Pocket Guide
to Sonography

D1478014

Pocket Guide to Sonography

Regina Swearengin, AAS, BS, RDMS
Department Chair
Sonography
Austin Community College
Austin, Texas

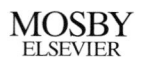

MOSBY
ELSEVIER

11830 Westline Industrial Drive
St. Louis, Missouri 63146

POCKET GUIDE TO SONOGRAPHY

ISBN: 978-0-323-04018-1

Library of Congress Control Number: 2007932284

Acquisitions Editor: Jeanne Wilke
Senior Developmental Editor: Linda Woodard
Publishing Services Manager: Patricia Tannian
Project Manager: Claire Kramer
Designer: Margaret Reid

Printed in China
Last digit is the print number: 9 8 7 6 5 4 3 2 1

Working together to grow
libraries in developing countries

www.elsevier.com | www.bookaid.org | www.sabre.org

ELSEVIER | BOOK AID International | Sabre Foundation

Reviewers

Sandra L. Hagen-Ansert, MS, RDMS, RDCS
Cardiology Department
Scripps Clinic Torrey Pines
La Jolla, California
Former Office Manager and Clinical Cardiac Sonographer
University Cardiology Associates, Medical University
 of South Carolina
Charleston, South Carolina

Moses M. Hdeib, MD, PhD, RDMS, RDCS, RVT
Clinical Associate Professor
Director, Diagnostic Medical Ultrasound Program
Director of Graduate Studies
University of Missouri–Columbia
Columbia, Missouri

Anthony Swartz, BS, RT(R), RDMS
Ob/Gyn Sonographer/Resident Ultrasound Education
 Coordinator
University of North Carolina
Chapel Hill, North Carolina

Kerry Weinberg, MPA, RT(R), RDMS, RDCS
Program Director
New York University
New York, New York

Bettye Wilson, MA-Ed, ARRT(R)(CT), RDMS, FASRT
Associate Professor
University of Alabama at Birmingham, School of Health
 Professions
Birmingham, Alabama

This pocket guide encompasses the abdominal, superficial, gynecologic, and obstetric specialty areas of sonography. The guide is designed to be a resource for practicing sonographers, especially entry-level sonographers who may need clarification or more information about sonographic findings, applicable measurements, or related disease processes encountered during the sonographic examination.

It is difficult for a sonographer to stop scanning to research unusual or unfamiliar findings using a variety of resources. This pocket guide is intended to provide a single point of reference that can be quickly used by the sonographer during the examination; however, this guide does not replace textbooks and other in-depth resources.

Student sonographers and experienced sonographers can benefit from this pocket guide. Student sonographers can find assistance with organizing the confusing landscape of sonographic findings/appearances, correlating the clinical presentation with the sonographic findings, and developing the critical thinking skills needed as a professional sonographer. Experienced sonographers who work in a specific type of practice (for example, obstetrics) sometimes need assistance if they are required to perform other types of studies; this pocket guide can serve as a refresher in those cases.

The sonographer must correctly interpret and document sonographic appearances seen on the monitor in order for the patient to receive the highest quality of care. The format of this pocket guide allows the sonographer to look up a description that matches sonographic findings, to correlate the patient's clinical presentation with the visual information, and to either reinforce or correct decisions made about the examination. In cases in which the ultrasound image is unfamiliar or confusing, the pocket guide can assist the sonographer in the performance of a thorough examination.

Multiple, well-known, highly regarded, and current resources have been used to summarize available information in this pocket guide. Inclusion of every sonographic appearance and disease state is not possible or feasible.

Content and Organization

This pocket guide is composed of chapters that are tabbed according to the topic of the chapter (e.g., Biliary System). Each chapter includes a section with basic information for each organ (patient preparation, specific equipment and technical factors, imaging protocol, normal variants, sonographic measurements, and common anomalies [when applicable]) and a table of Sonographic Findings, Clinical Presentation, Differential Diagnosis, and Next Step.

Fundamentals

"Fundamentals" (Chapter 1) includes general information and tips about patient preparation, technical factors, general protocols and procedures, ergonomics, and terminology. Specific information for patient preparation, technical settings, protocols, and measurements are included in the organ chapters.

Tables

The Sonographic Findings are generally arranged from most common to least common; therefore the Differential Diagnosis column content *will not* be in alphabetical order. The Sonographic Findings column lists the most common finding first and may list additional or possible other findings when appropriate. Because of the variety of sonographic appearances that may be seen in the same disease process, several rows listing the same initial sonographic appearance with slight to significant variations in findings may be used.

The Clinical Presentation column includes patient symptoms and signs and pertinent abnormal lab values (normal lab values are found in Appendix C) associated with the most common disease process. Occasionally, the clinical presentation includes lab values that might be seen if there is a complication (such as hemorrhage) associated with the disease process.

The Differential Diagnosis column lists disease processes in order of the most to least likely to occur, with the most common disease listed first and separate from the rest. Occasionally a short definition or explanation may be shown with a disease process.

The Next Step is a column that includes related pathologic conditions, suggestions for scanning other areas, organs or vessels, reminders about pitfalls encountered with the Sonographic Findings or Differential Diagnosis, and related imaging examinations and other testing. The Next Step is not intended to supersede the protocols of an institution but instead should serve to guide the sonographer in pursuing a thorough examination. As with all areas of this pocket guide, information in the Next Step has been garnered from published resources and from sonographer experiences that support the published material. Basic scanning protocols and procedures,

correlation of sonographic findings with clinical presentation, and differential diagnosis are integral to the practice of a professional sonographer, and the Next Step is the area that sets sonography apart from other imaging modalities and practices.

Appendixes

Several appendixes that provide specific references for protocols, measurements, normal lab values, and Doppler flow characteristics are included.

Glossary

The glossary lists symbols and abbreviations used in the *Pocket Guide to Sonography.*

Bibliography

All resources are listed in alphabetical order.

Each and every sonographer, colleague, physician, and student that I have been privileged to know, learn from, teach, and work alongside led to the creation of this book. I especially appreciate the information and encouragement I received from sonographers and doctors at Doctor's North and West Hospitals, Columbus, Ohio; Akron Children's Hospital; Barberton Citizens Hospital, Barberton, Ohio; and in Austin, Texas. In addition, the Austin Community College Diagnostic Medical Sonography Class of 2006 is acknowledged for their input and inspiration for this book.

Acknowledgments

Contents

Chapter 1 Fundamentals

Sonographers must have an in-depth understanding of the all facets of ultrasound imaging to perform examinations efficiently and accurately. The sonographic examination is not a collection of "pictures." It is the result of a thorough, active evaluation of the region of interest documented by images selected to best represent that evaluation. The sonographer uses the fundamentals of sonography in addition to specific or advanced techniques to produce a diagnostic-quality examination. Appropriate protocols, procedures, technical factors, ergonomics, and terminology must be used at all times.

Patient Preparation

Patient preparation (prep) instructions for each type of sonographic examination are available from a variety of publications (see Appendix A). Here are some tips on patient prep:

Upper abdomen

- Examinations performed later than the early morning may be significantly compromised by increasing amounts of air in the bowel (some air is swallowed while talking).

- Diabetic patients should be done as early in the day as possible; the patient may need to eat and drink immediately after the scan is completed, even while still in the examination room.
- Abdomen and pelvis sonograms scheduled for the same patient on the same day: it is extremely important that the patient understand the two separate preparations (if the full urinary bladder prep is used) and that the examinations may not be completed in one appointment time.

Gallbladder

- If the patient did not follow the fasting prep instructions the result may be a nondiagnostic examination that must be repeated.
- Smoking can cause the gallbladder to contract even when the patient has fasted.

Renal/urinary system

- The hydration level of the patient can affect the sonographic appearance of the kidneys (the renal medulla is generally more visible when the patient is hydrated).

- If the patient is fasting, visualization of urine jets in the bladder may be difficult or impossible.
- Overhydration of the patient (seen with the full urinary bladder prep) may lead to findings of pseudo or transient hydronephrosis.

Pelvis (female)

- Some protocols call for performing the transabdominal scan using whatever fluid is in the bladder at that time and then performing an endovaginal scan (after the patient voids) to obtain the required images.

Pregnancy

- The full urinary bladder examination may improve visualization of the lower uterine segment but may also create or mask cervical or placenta conditions. Using whatever fluid is in the urinary bladder may be more beneficial.

Pediatric patient

- Sonograms generally follow the same preparations as adult examinations, but fasting time is reduced or may not be needed.

- An emergency sonogram examination for any organ, structure, or area does not require any patient preparation.

Equipment and Technical Factors

The sonographer should have an in-depth knowledge of ultrasound physics and instrumentation (equipment hardware and software) to efficiently and accurately operate the ultrasound unit. Consult the technical publication(s) supplied with the unit or contact the applications support provided by the equipment manufacturer for clarification or instruction on equipment usage. Here are some tips regarding equipment and technical factors:

- The ultrasound unit should have appropriate software and transducers for all the applications performed in a clinical setting.

Fundamentals

- A single examination may require different types of transducers (sector, curved linear, etc.) to adequately evaluate the organ of interest.
- Curved linear transducers work well for many types of upper abdominal examinations, but a vector transducer can use the intercostal spaces to avoid rib artifacts and increase sound beam access to the liver, spleen, and kidneys (depending on the patient's body habitus).
- Equipment controls: choose the appropriate preset (manufacturer or user installed) for the examination type or area of interest; the sonographer should not expect the presets to fit in all scanning situations.
- Mechanical Index (MI) and Thermal Index (TI) settings must comply with the ALARA (as low as reasonably achievable) principle for all examinations (especially critical in pediatric and obstetrical studies).
- Overall gain, time gain compensation, depth, and focal zone placement(s) should be adjusted during the examination to ensure optimal imaging. Some organs/structures will require many readjustments of these settings because of organ/structure location, size, or region of interest within the organ/structure.
- It is impossible to establish standard settings for any sonogram because each patient's body habitus/organ orientation, amount and type of adipose tissue; normal variants, anomalies, and sonographic appearance of disease are unique to that individual.
- The use of harmonics will not always allow for easier scanning of patients or improve diagnostic quality of images (e.g., harmonics can reduce the visualization of actual echoes within a cyst). The sonographer should scan by using both conventional and harmonic imaging and select the most appropriate image.
- Spectral Doppler imaging should not be used for locating or documenting the embryonic heart rate because of the high intensities focused on the developing heart. If the embryonic heart is difficult to locate with two-dimensional or M-mode imaging,

power or color Doppler imaging can assist in the location of the heart and then M-mode imaging used to document the heart rate.
- Use of advanced imaging techniques such as three- or four-dimensional imaging and image compounding requires advanced scanning skill to be useful during the sonographic examination.

Imaging Protocol and Procedures

Detailed protocols and procedures are available for each type of examination (see Appendix C). Here are some tips regarding protocols and procedures:
- Written policies, protocols, and procedures should be created with input from sonographers and interpreting physicians. This document serves as a point of reference for the sonographer's clinical practice.
- All sonographers should comply with written policies, protocols, and procedures for all examinations to ensure consistency and high-quality patient care. Standard Precautions should be followed for all patients and exams.

- Overview scanning through the region of interest alerts the sonographer to the presence of technical difficulties, anomalies, and normal variants. The sonographer should correlate the sonogram with pertinent related imaging studies.
- A detailed scan through of the organ or region of interest increases the sonographer's ability to detect subtle changes in echogenicity, echotexture, organ/structure displacement, or other signs of abnormality.
- Appropriate settings for technical controls can be evaluated and adjusted during the overview scan or scan through.
- A logical pattern/method for image acquisition is more efficient and reproducible.
- Examination protocol or procedures may be adjusted during the examination on the basis of the sonographer's judgment of the scanning situation.
- Departmental procedures should specify what measurements are required for each organ/structure; use standard published resources for measurement criteria (see Appendix B).
- Departmental policies should specify a standard and efficient (clear and concise) image-labeling format.

- Labels should not cover the image or measurement readouts.
- Labels must be visible after the image is recorded.

Upper abdomen

- Repeated deep breathing may compromise the examination. Have the patient breathe in through the nose and not the mouth.
- The "belly out" technique or simply having the patient suspend respiration does not add air into the bowel.
- Perform the examination with the patient in a semi-Fowler or slight reverse-Trendelenburg position to place more of the liver anterior to the pancreas.

Renal/urinary system

- In cases of suspected pseudo or transient hydronephrosis, reimage the kidneys after the patient voids.
- The urinary bladder with documentation of urine jets, if possible, should be included to thoroughly evaluate the urinary system.

Pelvis (female)

- Transabdominal imaging: The bladder may be overly distended, distorting the anatomy requiring the patient to partially void.

Pregnancy

- Some protocols require documenting urinary bladder fullness followed by endovaginal imaging to evaluate cervical length or placenta location.
- Transperineal scanning can also be used to evaluate the lower uterine segment, placental location, and cervical length.

Ergonomics

Information and assistance with sonographer ergonomics is available from a variety of sources. Here are some reminders/tips for good ergonomics:

- Good ergonomic principles must be learned, adopted, and practiced. Occasions where ergonomic scanning is not possible should be infrequent.

- No one will care about the sonographer's health and well-being more than the sonographer himself/herself.
- Protection from injury to the sonographer is just as important as protecting the patient from injury during the sonogram...don't create another patient!
- Emphasis on speedy scanning over efficient and accurate scanning can cause a decrease in a sonographer's career longevity and health.
- Professionals use professional "tools." The professional sonographer operates the ultrasound equipment correctly and uses ancillary devices to obtain the best quality examination.
- Ultrasound imaging does have limitations, which the sonographer should not try to circumvent by using injury-causing scanning techniques.

Imaging Terminology

Information on sonographic terminology (physics and imaging terms) can be found in a variety of resources; however, agreement on imaging terms is not universal. Here are some reminders about imaging terms:

- Anechoic means that no echoes were returned.
- Terms that describe and quantify echogenicity are relative; a structure is more or less echogenic than another structure.
- Terms that describe echotexture should be used.
  - Homogeneous is an even or smooth texture.
  - Heterogeneous is an uneven or variable texture.
  - Coarse is a slightly less homogeneous texture.
- Borders of a structure can be described as well-defined, smooth, irregular, or infiltrating.
- Loculated describes septa within a structure (thin, thick).
- Increased through transmission or acoustic enhancement describes some degree of increased echogenicity immediately posterior to a structure caused by lack of attenuation of sound (fluid or fluid-filled structure).
- Decreased through transmission or acoustic attenuation results in less echogenicity posterior to a solid structure.
- Some use the terms sonolucent or echolucent instead of anechoic.
- Some use the terms sonodense or echodense instead of hyperechoic.

ABDOMEN

Patient Preparation

- Patients should fast for 6 to 12 hours; emergency examinations may be done with or without fasting.

Equipment and Technical Factors

- A curved linear multihertz transducer is preferred; a sector/vector transducer may be required for intercostal imaging.
- Decrease the dynamic range to produce higher contrast in images of the gallbladder and ducts; use of harmonics is recommended.
- Color Doppler imaging can be used to distinguish vascular from nonvascular structures, especially in cases where hepatic artery or bile duct variants are present.

Imaging Protocol

Minimum documentation images for the gallbladder

- Longitudinal axis images of the medial, mid, and lateral portions.
- Transverse axis images of the proximal (neck), mid (body), and distal (fundus).
- Measure anterior gallbladder wall in a longitudinal or transverse midgallbladder image; any region of suspected wall thickening should be measured.
- At least two of the following patient positions must be used: supine, left lateral decubitus, upright/semiupright, or prone. Other positions may be helpful.

Minimum documentation images for the extrahepatic bile duct

- Longitudinal images of the extrahepatic bile duct proximal, mid, and distal with lumen measurements or measurement at largest diameter. Transverse axis image(s) of the portal triad or common bile duct at the head of pancreas should be included.

Normal Variants

- Phrygian cap (fundus of gallbladder): does not change with patient position.

- Hartmann's pouch (neck of gallbladder): does not change with patient position.
- Junctional gallbladder fold: with change in patient position, fold may or may not persist.
- Variation of shape: gallbladder is more round or elongated than oval/pear shaped.
- Variations in the location where the cystic duct joins with the common hepatic duct and accessory hepatic ducts may be seen.

Sonographic Measurements

- Gallbladder: <4.0 cm in anteroposterior and transverse and <8.0–12.0 cm longitudinal; wall thickness <3.0 mm anteroposterior.
- Biliary ducts
  Common hepatic duct: <4.0 mm
  Common bile duct, <65 years of age: 6.0–7.0 mm
  Common bile duct, >65 years of age: 10.0 mm
  Post cholecystectomy: 6.0–11.0 mm

Biliary System

Sonographic Finding(s)	Clinical Presentation	Differential Diagnosis	Next Step
Low-level echoes within GB May see layering effect May appear as "mass"	Asymptomatic *or* Symptoms and laboratory values as seen in acute cholecystitis Prolonged fasting state	Sludge/viscid bile	May be transient because of the patient's fasting state or related to gallbladder disease
Echogenic, mobile structure(s) with shadowing within GB May "layer"	Asymptomatic *or* right upper quadrant pain Nausea Vomiting Positive Murphy's sign Labs: elevated direct bilirubin and LFTs	Cholelithiasis	Ensure that a high-frequency and focal zone is properly placed Color Doppler imaging may be used to demonstrate the "twinkle" sign in the presence of tiny stones Evaluate for hepatic biliary obstruction, pancreatitis

GB wall thickening, possible gallstone(s), with/without pericholecystic fluid	Possible: RUQ pain Nausea Vomiting Positive Murphy's sign Fever Labs: elevated direct bilirubin with obstruction	Cholelithiasis with acute cholecystitis	Associated with biliary obstruction and pancreatitis, especially when tiny/small gallstones are present Increased flow may be noted in the cystic artery
Wall is uniformly thickened, with/without pericholecystic fluid	Sudden onset of RUQ pain, possibly radiating to right shoulder or back Fever Nausea Vomiting Positive Murphy's sign Labs: elevated LFTs, serum amylase Leukocytosis	Acute cholecystitis Hepatitis (marked thickening) AIDS cholangiopathy Sclerosing cholangitis	Commonly associated with cholelithiasis

continued

Biliary System—*cont'd*

Sonographic Finding(s)	Clinical Presentation	Differential Diagnosis	Next Step
Wall is uniformly thickened and the gallbladder is small despite patient fasting	Transient RUQ pain for 6 months or greater Dyspepsia Fat intolerance Flatulence Nausea Vomiting Labs: elevated LFTs and serum amylase	Chronic cholecystitis	Commonly associated with cholelithiasis Disease may be noted in the liver, bile ducts, and pancreas

Distended gallbladder not seen; echogenic area with shadowing noted in gallbladder fossa area
WES sign
	Chronic symptoms:
	  Bloating
	  Belching
	  Food avoidance
	  RUQ pain
	Negative
	Murphy's sign
		Chronic cholelithiasis/ cholecystitis
		Collapsed/nondistended GB
		Loop of bowel
			Associated with biliary obstruction or pancreatitis

	Labs: elevated direct bilirubin with obstruction Asymptomatic patient did not fast	Collapsed/nondistended GB versus loop of bowel	Nondiagnostic study; rescan after fasting prep
Wall is uniformly thickened GB is normal sized Dilated hepatic veins and IVC (CHF)	Possible abdominal swelling Soft tissue edema Liver enlargement RUQ pain Labs: associated with underlying disease process(es) Hypoproteinemia Hypoalbuminemia	Noninflammatory wall thickening	Associated with ascites, carcinoma, cirrhosis, sepsis, renal disease, AIDS, pancreatitis, CHF Concurrent GB disease possible

continued

Biliary System—*cont'd*

Sonographic Finding(s)	Clinical Presentation	Differential Diagnosis	Next Step
Wall is thickened with areas of decreased echogenicity Ascites may be noted	Nausea Flatulence Light-colored stool Weakness Abdominal pain Varicosities Spider angiomas Labs: abnormal LFTs	GB varices	Cause: portal hypertension Color Doppler imaging to evaluate flow in GB wall
Small, nonmobile mass(es) projecting into GB lumen	Asymptomatic *or* RUQ pain	Polyp(s) Hyperplastic cholecystosis Cholesterolosis	Generally an incidental finding Polyp enlargement may indicate malignancy

Wall is irregularly or segmentally thickened; echogenic foci or anechoic areas noted in the wall "Comet-tail" or shadowing artifact(s) may be seen arising from GB wall	Asymptomatic *or* RUQ pain	Hyperplastic cholecystosis Cholesterolosis Adenomyomatosis	Mimics emphysematous cholecystitis X-ray/CT to differentiate air from cholesterol crystals
Massive thickening and striation of GB wall, possible gallstone(s), with/without pericholecystic fluid	History of acute cholecystitis Fever Generalized abdominal pain Labs: elevated LFTs, serum amylase, leukocytosis	Gangrenous cholecystitis	Gangrene may extend beyond GB Gallbladder/duodenal fistula may be present

continued

Biliary System—*cont'd*

Sonographic Finding(s)	Clinical Presentation	Differential Diagnosis	Next Step
Focal irregular thickening of GB wall, debris within GB, and pericholecystic fluid	History of acute cholecystitis Labs: leukocytosis, elevated ALP	Empyema of GB	
Air in GB wall with/without gallstones	RUQ pain Fever History of diabetes Labs: elevated bilirubin, ALP	Emphysematous Cholecystitis	Associated with cholelithiasis, GB gangrene and rupture, pneumobilia
Echogenic nonmobile structure(s), shadowing within GB; possible wall thickening	RUQ pain Nausea Vomiting Positive Murphy's sign Fever Labs: elevated direct bilirubin	Impacted gallstone with/without cholecystitis	Impacted gallstone may cause development of fistula between GB and duodenum

Mass filling or completely filling GB Gallstones Possible porcelain GB Ascites may be noted	Weight loss Anorexia RUQ pain Jaundice Nausea Vomiting Hepatomegaly Labs: elevated direct bilirubin with obstruction	Carcinoma of GB Tumefactive sludge Inflammatory wall thickening Polyps Focal adenomyomatosis	Symptoms noted with advanced disease Metastases to liver, bile ducts, vessels, lymph nodes, peritoneal cavity
Segmental or completely echogenic GB wall—echogenic "arc" with shadow Gallstones possible	Asymptomatic May relate to history of cholecystitis	Porcelain GB WES gallbladder Emphysematous GB	Some association with GB carcinoma

Biliary System—*cont'd*

Sonographic Finding(s)	Clinical Presentation	Differential Diagnosis	Next Step
Prominent CBD (internal lumen >7.0 mm) With/without prominent CHD (internal lumen >4.0 mm)	Advanced patient age or postcholecystectomy RUQ pain Labs: elevated direct bilirubin with obstruction	Ectasia of bile duct from advanced patient age Development of postsurgical bile duct strictures	Demonstrate termination of duct if stricture is suspected
Dilated CBD (internal lumen >7.0 mm); calculus within duct or at duct termination (may be multiple) With/without dilated CHD (internal lumen >4.0 mm) With/without intrahepatic tubular structures with jagged branching pattern (parallel-channel sign; acoustic enhancement)	Severe RUQ pain Jaundice Presurgical or postsurgical patient Labs: elevated direct bilirubin, ALP	Choledocholithiasis	Gallstones may be noted; stones may be extremely small or tiny Gallstones may reflux into bile duct during or after cholecystectomy

Dilated CBD (internal lumen >7.0 mm); duct terminates; no calculus is seen With/without dilated CHD (internal lumen >4 .0 mm) With/without dilated intrahepatic ducts GB enlargement	Possible RUQ pain Jaundice with/without pain Labs: elevated direct bilirubin, amylase, lipase	Enlargement of head of pancreas from mass or pancreatitis	Demonstrate superior and inferior borders of pancreatic head in longitudinal axis
Dilated CHD (internal lumen >4.0 mm) with/without dilated intrahepatic ducts "Central dot" sign may be seen Calcification in cystic duct	Jaundice Labs: elevated direct bilirubin with obstruction	Mirizzi syndrome (cystic duct stone compressing CHD) Cholangitis	Cholelithiasis or choledolithiasis may be present

continued

Biliary System—*cont'd*

Sonographic Finding(s)	Clinical Presentation	Differential Diagnosis	Next Step
Mass at juncture of right and left hepatic ducts causing dilated intrahepatic ducts (parallel-channel sign, acoustic enhancement) May appear to be near porta hepatis	RUQ pain Anorexia Weight loss Jaundice Labs: elevated direct bilirubin, ALP, ALT, AST	Klatskin tumor (carcinoma at hepatic duct juncture) Lymphadenopathy	Lymphadenopathy may demonstrate as multiple nodes
Dilated bile duct(s) with/without enlargement of GB wall	Jaundice Labs: elevated LFTs, direct bilirubin if obstruction present	Cholangitis (associated with bacterial infection or biliary obstruction) AIDS cholangitis	AIDS cholangitis may progress to sclerosing cholangitis
Massively dilated bile ducts without evidence of stones Large, palpable GB may be noted	Fever RUQ/epigastric pain Jaundice	Oriental (recurrent pyogenic) cholangitis Biliary obstruction	Associated with bile duct strictures, bacterial infection in bile, and parasites in ducts

Air within biliary system may be seen	Labs: markedly elevated direct bilirubin, ALP; elevated WBC, AST, ALT	Caroli disease	
Thickened, echogenic intrahepatic or extrahepatic bile duct walls	Fever RUQ/epigastric pain Jaundice History of ulcerative colitis Labs: markedly elevated direct bilirubin and ALP; elevated WBC, AST, ALT	Sclerosing cholangitis	Associated with congenital or acquired strictures, parasitic infestation, and infection caused by biliary calculi May mimic pneumobilia or arteriosclerosis
Intrahepatic tubular structures with jagged branching pattern (parallel-channel sign, acoustic enhancement) Mass(es) within ducts, most often in CBD or CHD	Jaundice Pruritus RUQ pain Biliary colic Weight loss Nausea	Cholangiocarcinoma	Associated with pancreatic carcinoma Cholelithiasis may be noted

continued

Biliary System—*cont'd*

Sonographic Finding(s)	Clinical Presentation	Differential Diagnosis	Next Step
Dilation of pancreatic duct Enlarged liver and ascites	Vomiting Labs: elevated direct bilirubin, ALP, AST		
Multiple cystic structures within liver	"Crampy" pain Intermittent jaundice Fever Labs: elevated LFT	Caroli disease (cystic dilation of intrahepatic bile ducts) Liver cysts Intrahepatic ducts	Complications: biliary stasis and obstruction, cholangitis, liver abscess, hepatic fibrosis Kidney cystic disease may be present
Intrahepatic linear hyperechoic structures with comet tail artifact or shadowing Hyperechoic linear structures seem to move with change in patient position	Recent bile duct surgery or ERCP History of cholangitis Labs: abnormal LFTs, amylase, lipase	Pneumobilia Choledocholithiasis Arterial calcifications	Plain film x-ray or CT may be needed to differentiate air from arterial calcifications Pancreatitis may be present

Cystic mass in porta hepatis	Jaundice RUQ pain Palpable mass Fever Labs: elevated direct bilirubin, WBC	Choledochal cyst Duplicated GB	Document GB separate from abnormal CBD

Patient Preparation

- Fasting is not required if only the liver is to be evaluated; however, the gallbladder and extrahepatic bile ducts (fasting examinations) are usually included in most evaluations of the liver.

Equipment and Technical Factors

- Because of the depth and breath of the liver, multiple transducer types (sector, vector, curved linear) may be used to thoroughly evaluate the liver. Use of high frequencies to image the anterior surface and left lobe of the liver is recommended. Use of lower frequencies to image the right lobe and diaphragm may be required.
- Technical settings should ensure that the liver parenchyma is a homogenous, midlevel shade of gray with anechoic blood vessels and hyperechoic ligaments, diaphragm, and blood vessel walls.

Imaging Protocol

- Longitudinal and transverse axis images should be recorded of the functional lobar anatomy: left, right, and caudate lobes. Include all surfaces of the liver, the porta hepatic, hepatic veins, portal veins, and the ligaments, fossa, and fissures.
- Images should be recorded in an efficient, logical, and sequential manner.
- Transverse axis image(s) of the portal triad at the porta hepatis should be included.
- Images may be labeled as Couinaud segments I–VIII as required (surgical resections, transplants).
- Color Doppler imaging may confirm flow in suspected vessels or the hepatic and portal veins and hepatic artery.

Variants

- Variations in liver shape and overall size may be noted, including Reidel's lobe and a small left lobe.

Sonographic Measurements (Normal Limits)

- Cranial to caudal (diaphragm to tip of right lobe) along the midclavicular line: 15.0 cm
- Main portal vein diameter: 13.0 mm
- Other measurements may be performed (may be difficult):
  Anterior to posterior through the right lobe: 10.0–21.0 cm
  Transverse lateral left lobe through lateral right lobe: 20.0–36.0 cm
- Liver volume: $133.2 + 0.422(CC \times AP \times LL)$
- Right lobe to caudate lobe ratio (from transverse image): diameter of caudate lobe (A) divided by diameter of the right lobe (B); a ratio >0.65 may indicate cirrhosis.

Liver

Sonographic Finding(s)	Clinical Presentation	Differential Diagnosis	Next Step

Liver measures >15.0 cm along midclavicular line *or*
 Extension of right lobe inferior to lower pole of kidney; inferior tip of right lobe may be rounded
 Left lobe may extend into LUQ
	Asymptomatic *or*
	 Symptoms may be associated with a variety of liver disease states
	 Labs: normal to elevated LFT
		Hepatomegaly is associated with a variety of diffuse disease processes:
		   Early cirrhosis
		   Anemia
		   Congestive heart failure
		   Portal hypertension
		   Fatty infiltration
		   Hepatitis
		 Normal variant or the result of patient's body habitus
			Evidence of disease may be subtle
			 May be caused by multiple focal disease: cyst, neoplasm, metastases, abscess
			 Splenomegaly may be present

Increased echogenicity of liver (mild to significant) with decreased visualization of liver landmarks
Mild to severe attenuation of sound
Diaphragm difficult to visualize
	Usually asymptomatic
	Possible jaundice, nausea and vomiting, abdominal tenderness/pain
	Labs: normal to elevated LFT
		Fatty infiltration
		Cirrhosis
		Hepatitis
		Metastatic disease
			Associated with:
			  ETOH abuse
			  Obesity
			  Pregnancy
			  Severe hepatitis
			  Steroid use
			  Chemotherapy
			  Diabetes
			  Glycogen storage disease
			Lower transducer frequencies and a variety of scan planes should be used
			Degree of fatty infiltration may be graded (1–3)

continued

Liver—*cont'd*

Sonographic Finding(s)	Clinical Presentation	Differential Diagnosis	Next Step
Patchy area of increased echogenicity near porta hepatis; may be fan shaped, angular, or band shaped No mass effect demonstrated with 2D or color Doppler imaging	Asymptomatic Labs: normal LFT	Focal fatty infiltration	Opposite of focal fatty sparing
Large liver with increased echogenicity throughout (possibly very echogenic) with area of lesser echogenicity anterior to right portal vein, near porta hepatis or posterior left lobe May at first appear as a "mass"; however, no mass effect is noted	Usually asymptomatic Labs: normal to elevated LFT	Focal fatty sparing	Opposite of focal fatty infiltration

Normal to hypoechoic liver echogenicity with or without hepatosplenomegaly Prominent portal vein walls may be noted ("starry-sky" appearance) Gallbladder wall thickening may be noted	Flu-like symptoms GI complaints Loss of appetite Low-grade fever Fatigue RUQ pain, jaundice Labs: elevated bilirubin, LDH, ALT, AST, leukopenia	Acute hepatitis: viral (mononucleosis) amebiasis, chemical or drug toxicity	The patient may not be diagnosed with hepatitis before the sonogram May mimic fatty liver
Normal-sized liver with increased echogenicity (may be brighter than fatty liver) Coarse/heterogenous appearance of liver texture; may be focal or patchy Some attenuation of sound but not as great as fatty liver Decreased brightness of the portal triads	Fatigue Nausea Anorexia Weight loss Jaundice Tremors Varicosities Dark urine Labs: elevated LFT, leukopenia, decreased BUN	Chronic hepatitis: all types except A	Symptoms for 6 months or more May mimic cirrhosis or fatty liver Portal hypertension may be present

continued

Liver—*cont'd*

Sonographic Finding(s)	Clinical Presentation	Differential Diagnosis	Next Step
Echogenic mass(es), homogeneous and well defined Round, oval, or lobulated; usually <3.0 cm Posterior enhancement may be noted	Commonly asymptomatic female patient Labs: normal LFT	Typical hemangioma HCC Adenoma Metastasis FNH	Use of power Doppler imaging may demonstrate flow within hemangioma
Hypoechoic mass or mass with hypoechoic center (reverse target) Variable echogenicity Posterior enhancement or calcifications may be noted	Commonly asymptomatic female patient Pregnancy RUQ pain Labs: normal LFT; decreased hematocrit with hemorrhage	Atypical hemangioma HCC Adenoma Metastasis FNH	Use of power Doppler imaging may demonstrate flow within hemangioma Variable echogenicity depends on amount of fibrosis and degeneration

Cystic structure with anechoic lumen; round or oval Increased through transmission Well-defined, thin walls	Asymptomatic May cause pain when large Labs: normal to elevated LFT	Congenital simple cyst(s)	Large cyst(s) can cause pain or mass effect within the liver
Cystic structure with internal echoes; round or oval Septations, solid elements, or calcification may be noted Increased through transmission Well-defined thick wall	Asymptomatic Possible hepatomegaly and jaundice Labs: normal to elevated LFT	Complex cyst(s) (infection or hemorrhage within a simple cyst) Necrotic tumor Hematoma Abscess Echinococcal cyst	Large cyst(s) can cause pain or mass effect within liver
Well-defined mass(es): echogenic central area with hypoechoic peripheral halo (target lesions)	Asymptomatic *or* Jaundice Pain Weight loss	Metastatic disease Hematoma Hepatoma FNH	Investigate portal and hepatic veins for tumor extension or thrombus development *continued*

Liver—*cont'd*

Sonographic Finding(s)	Clinical Presentation	Differential Diagnosis	Next Step
	Anorexia Hepatomegaly History of malignancy especially breast, lung, and colon Labs: abnormal LFT	Adenoma Abscess Hydatid cyst Hemangioma Granulomatous disease	Use high-frequency transducer to evaluate periphery of the liver, especially in diffuse-appearing disease

Increased echogenicity of liver with possible hepatomegaly
Coarsening of liver echotexture
Sound attenuation but not as great as fatty liver; decreased visualization of vascular structures
Ascites
	Asymptomatic *or*
	Nausea
	Anorexia
	Weight loss
	Flatulence
	Weakness
	Abdominal pain
	Varicosities
	Labs: elevated LFT, leukopenia
		Acute cirrhosis
		Fatty liver
		Hepatitis
			Associated with:
			  ETOH abuse
			  Hepatitis
			  Biliary disease
			  Metabolic disease
			  Pancreatitis
			Early portal hypertension may be present

Small liver size with nodular border and heterogenous echo texture Caudate lobe enlargement (caudate/right lobe ratio of >0.65) Portal hypertension, varices, and ascites may be noted	Nausea Anorexia Weight loss Flatulence Weakness Abdominal pain Varicosities Spider angiomas Labs: elevated LFT, leukopenia	Chronic cirrhosis Diffuse primary or metastatic carcinoma	Associated with increased incidence of HCC Use high frequency to evaluate for border nodularity
Hepatofugal flow in portal vein Enlarged vessel diameters in portal venous system Varices and ascites may be noted Increased flow in hepatic artery may be noted	History of cirrhosis, use of oral contraceptives, pancreatitis, splenectomy, coagulopathy, sclerosing cholangitis Acute onset of Budd-Chiari syndrome or congestive heart failure Hemoptysis	Portal hypertension (intrahepatic, extrahepatic, hyperdynamic, or idiopathic cause)	In the presence of collaterals, portal system vessels may have normal diameters Document size and flow in hepatic artery Vessels may be occluded and appear anechoic with gray-scale imaging

continued

Liver—*cont'd*

Sonographic Finding(s)	Clinical Presentation	Differential Diagnosis	Next Step
	Jaundice Labs: abnormal values associated with primary etiology		

Nonvisualization of portal vein or echoes within portal vein
Dilated splenic and superior mesenteric vein proximal to the level of obstruction in portal vein
Ascites and splenomegaly are noted
Prominent periportal collaterals noted anterior to the portal vein (cavernous transformation)
	History of HCC, cirrhosis, pancreatic or GI cancer, or lymphoma
	Increasing abdominal girth
	Possible GI bleeding
	Labs: Abnormal lab values are associated with the underlying cause
		Portal vein thrombosis	Associated with:
			  Portal hypertension
			  Sepsis
			  Trauma
			  Cirrhosis
			  HCC
			Tumor invasion
			Requires combination of gray-scale and color Doppler imaging to confirm presence of intraluminal filling defects or absence of flow in the portal vein

Isoechoic mass in liver Possibly hypoechoic or hyperechoic	Asymptomatic *or* RUQ pain Use of oral contraceptives	FNH (congenital hepatocellular hyperplasia)	Possible concurrent adenoma Hemorrhage may cause pain and decreased hematocrit
Well-defined lesion, hyperechoic center with hypoechoic halo Mass that is isoechoic to the liver Hypoechoic mass(es) Brightly echogenic mass(es) Multiple ill-defined masses; may appear as diffuse heterogeneous parenchymal pattern Hypoechoic mass(es) with calcification Cystic mass(es) with thick walls	Asymptomatic *or* RUQ pain Use of oral contraceptives or steroids (males) History of von Gierke's disease Labs: normal LFT, decreased hematocrit with hemorrhage	Adenoma FNH Hepatoma Atypical hemangioma	Central echogenic area related to hemorrhage Rupture may lead to shock and hemoperitoneum Low risk of malignancy

continued

Liver—*cont'd*

Sonographic Finding(s)	Clinical Presentation	Differential Diagnosis	Next Step
Large dominant lesion with/ without scattered smaller satellite lesions Variable echogenicity	Fever Cirrhosis Hepatomegaly Associated with cirrhosis, hepatitis B & C, ofloxacin, carcinogens Labs: abnormal LFT, elevated AFP	HCC Hepatoma	Use high frequency to evaluate the periphery of liver
Complex, space-occupying mass with thick, irregular walls, septations, or debris Possible presence of air (increased echogenicity with shadowing)	Fever, RUQ pain Nausea Vomiting Anorexia Fatigue Diarrhea	Abscess: pyogenic (bacterial) amebic (parasitic) fungal	Use high-frequency transducer to evaluate the periphery of the liver Fluid may be found in potential spaces

	Clinical Findings	Differential Diagnosis	Comments
	Jaundice Hepatomegaly Anemia Asymptomatic (amebic) Labs: elevated WBC, abnormal LFT, RBC	Hematoma Jaundice Hemorrhagic cyst/tumor Necrotic tumor Echinococcal cyst	Color Doppler imaging may depict flow in abscess wall
Echogenic to cystic "mass" noted at periphery of liver (subcapsular) or intraparenchymal Possible hepatomegaly	RUQ pain Fever Hypotension History of: trauma, neoplasm, or HELLP syndrome Labs: decreased hematocrit	Hematoma Abscess Complex mass	Change in sonographic appearance over time; serial sonograms may be necessary

continued

Liver—*cont'd*

Sonographic Finding(s)	Clinical Presentation	Differential Diagnosis	Next Step
Multiple hypoechoic masses with echogenic center; "wheel within wheel"/ bull's-eye lesions	Immunocompromised patient	Hepatic candidiasis Abscess Echinococcal cyst Metastases	Calcifications may be noted
Multiple echogenic foci diffusely scattered through the parenchyma	History of: *Pneumocystis carinii*, cytomegalovirus, histoplasmosis	Granulomatous disease (granulomas that demonstrate calcification) Abscess(es)	Evaluate the spleen for presence of calcifications
Hepatomegaly with normal or diffuse echogenicity changes	FUO Anemia Night sweats Weakness	Hodgkin's lymphoma	May mimic multifocal hepatoma or metastases May involve: Spleen

	Malaise
	Weight loss
	Enlarged nontender lymph
	  nodes
	Abdominal mass
	Labs: abnormal LFT, RBC;
	  leukocytosis
			Kidneys
			Retroperitoneum
			Testes

Hepatomegaly with
  hypoechoic to anechoic
  lesions
Mass(es) may displace
  organs or great vessels
	Night sweats
	Weakness
	Malaise
	Weight loss
	Enlarged nontender lymph
	  nodes
	Back pain
	Immunosuppressed patient
	Labs: abnormal LFT
		Non-Hodgkin's
		lymphoma
			May mimic neoplasm or
			  multifocal hepatoma
			May involve: spleen,
			  retroperitoneum, testes
			In children may be related
			  to neuroblastoma, Wilms'
			  tumor, and leukemia

continued

Liver—*cont'd*

Sonographic Finding(s)	Clinical Presentation	Differential Diagnosis	Next Step
Unable to demonstrate anechoic hepatic veins No flow in hepatic veins IVC or hepatic vein thrombus may be seen Large, hypoechoic caudate lobe Hepatomegaly Ascites	Abdominal pain Jaundice Use of oral contraceptives Pregnancy Trauma History of HCC, renal cell carcinoma, polycythemia vera, or sickle cell disease Labs: abnormal LFT	Budd-Chiari syndrome (thrombosis of hepatic veins) Idiopathic cirrhosis	Thrombosis may extend into the IVC Document caudate lobe/right lobe ratio (>0.65 is abnormal) Document features of portal hypertension
Large anechoic structure(s) with thick and irregular walls with/without low level echoes within	Hepatomegaly Pain Nausea RUQ pressure	Echinococcal (hydatid) cyst Polycystic disease Amebic abscess	Large cysts may rupture Cyst may cause vascular thrombosis and infarction

Possible presence of "daughter" cysts or cyst within cyst ("water lily" sign) Possible calcifications within walls	Jaundice Increased abdomen size Exposure to sheep herding or eating wild game Labs: elevated WBC	Pyogenic abscess

Patient Preparation

- Fasting for 6 to 12 hours; emergency examinations may be done without fasting.

Equipment and Technical Factors

- A curved linear multihertz transducer is preferred.
- The pancreas is more echogenic than the liver in the adult patient, and isoechoic to less echogenic in pediatric age groups; images should clearly demonstrate the relational vascular landmarks.
- The pancreas generally decreases in size and increases in echogenicity with age.
- Color Doppler imaging may be used to distinguish between a vessel and a bile duct.

Imaging Protocol

- Longitudinal axis images (transverse scan plane) through the head, neck, body and tail (if possible) should be obtained; these images will also include the great vessels, portal vein, and splenic vein, and artery.
- Transverse axis images (sagittal scan plane) of the head/uncinate process, neck, body, and tail should be obtained; these images will also include the great vessels, portal vein, and splenic vein and artery.
- The relationship of the CBD and pancreas head in longitudinal and transverse axes should be demonstrated.
- Measurements of the pancreas may be included; measurements must be done when pathology is detected.

- Semiupright to upright patient positions, "belly-out" breathing technique, or oral ingestion of water or contrast agent may improve visualization of the pancreas (water or contrast may be contraindicated in some patients).

Sonographic Measurements

Pancreas

Measurements are performed in the anterior to posterior dimension perpendicular to the longitudinal axis of the pancreas:

Head: <3.0 cm (range: 2.0–3.5 cm)
Neck: 1.0–2.0 cm
Body: <2.5 cm (range: 1.2–3 cm)
Tail: <2.5 cm (range: 1.0–2.8 cm)
- Length: 12–15 cm (generally not measured sonographically)
- Main pancreatic duct (MPD) lumen diameter: <2 mm

Pancreas

Sonographic Finding(s)	Clinical Presentation	Differential Diagnosis	Next Step
Patient is focally tender when scanning over a pancreas with normal sonographic appearance Pancreas less echogenic than normal for age Pancreas less echogenic than normal for age *and* demonstrates focal or diffuse enlargement (>3.0 cm AP head or tail) With or without MPD enlargement With or without pseudocyst formation	Pain (possibly severe) Fever Fatty stool History of ERCP or pancreatic cancer Labs: elevated serum amylase (within 24 h) and lipase (within 72–94 h), direct bilirubin, ALP, WBC Urine amylase elevates 6–10 days after symptoms; remains elevated longer	Acute pancreatitis	Commonly associated with gallstones No pressure when scanning the pancreas if pseudocyst is noted! Focal enlargement may be confused with pancreatic carcinoma

Focal or diffuse enlargement (possibly massive) with possible increased echogenicity (related to hemorrhage progression) CBD obstruction	Severe pain radiating to back Shock Ileus Hypotension History of excessive eating in one sitting or drinking alcoholic beverages Labs: decreased hematocrit and serum calcium level	Hemorrhagic or necrotizing pancreatitis Chronic hemorrhage	No pressure while scanning! Life-threatening sequel of pancreatitis! Fluid accumulation may be noted in retroperitoneum and flanks; Grey Turner sign (discoloration of flanks from pooling of blood)
Small, echogenic pancreas when age is considered Possible calcifications in pancreatic parenchyma or MPD With or without pancreatic pseudocyst noted Portal vein thrombosis	Increasing epigastric pain radiating to back GI complaints Weight loss Jaundice Fatty stool diabetes Labs: elevated serum amylase and lipase	Chronic pancreatitis Acute pancreatitis	Pancreatic duct may be mistaken for CBD May have acute superimposed on chronic pancreatitis No pressure when scanning the pancreas if pseudocyst is noted!

continued

Pancreas—*cont'd*

Sonographic Finding(s)	Clinical Presentation	Differential Diagnosis	Next Step
"Cyst" noted near the tail of the pancreas or lesser sac; patient has known pancreatitis Completely anechoic but without well-defined wall Possible thick wall Possible debris within structure Acoustic enhancement noted	Asymptomatic *or* Focal midepigastric tenderness Pain, possibly severe Fever Labs: elevated serum amylase, lipase, ALP	Pancreatic pseudocyst Fluid-filled cystadenoma True cyst of pancreas	No pressure when scanning! Evaluate the retroperitoneum and lesser sac for fluid (pancreatic fluid or blood) May require serial sonograms
Hypoechoic mass/area noted head of the pancreas Possible MPD or CBD dilation With or without an extremely large GB (Courvoisier GB) Possible ascites	Asymptomatic *or* Dull abdominal pain radiating to back Midepigastric pain Weight loss Painless jaundice Nausea	Carcinoma of the pancreas (95% are adenocarcinoma) Lymphoma	Evaluate the portal venous system and retroperitoneum for presence of disease Evaluate the superior and inferior dimensions for extension of the mass

	Vomiting History or diabetes Labs: Elevated bilirubin, ALP, amylase		Pancreatic adenocarcinoma can occur in other areas of the pancreas
Cysts in pancreas Cysts have irregular, lobulated, thick walls Calcifications may be noted	Epigastric pain Weight loss Palpable mass Jaundice Labs: elevated amylase	Cystadenoma Cystadenocarcinoma Pseudocyst Metastases	Patient may have concurrent disease: diabetes, choledocholithiasis, hypertension
Small hypoechoic mass in tail of pancreas	Palpable mass Sweating Insulin shock Dizziness Nausea/vomiting Labs: hyperinsulinism, hypoglycemia	Insulinoma Pancreatic carcinoma Lymphoma	Insulinomas may be solitary, multiple, or diffuse

Patient Preparation

- No preparation is required, although if it is included in a complete abdomen examination, the patient may be fasting.

Equipment and Technical Factors

- Curved linear multihertz transducer is needed; sector/vector transducer may be required for intercostal imaging.
- The spleen demonstrates a very homogenous echotexture and midlevel echogenicity that is isoechoic to hypoechoic to the liver; the blood vessels are generally only noted at the hilum.
- Color Doppler imaging may confirm the direction of flow in the splenic vessels.

Imaging Protocol

- A variety of transducer placements (scan planes) may be used to obtain diagnostic images of the spleen; therefore, each image must be labeled accurately for scan plane and anatomy demonstrated.
  - Longitudinal axis images through the medial, mid (hilum), and lateral aspects of the spleen are obtained; if the coronal plane is used, then the anterior, mid, and inferior aspects are documented.
  - Transverse axis images through the superior, mid (hilum), and inferior aspects of the spleen are obtained; the transverse lateral scan plane may be used to obtain these images.

- The relationship of the spleen with the surrounding anatomy should be documented; echogenicity comparison with the left kidney should be performed.

Sonographic Measurements

The spleen is variable in shape.

- Length: <13 cm as measured from superior to inferior pole; 7.0–9.0 cm if measured from the diaphragm to inferior tip (range 5.5–14.0 cm)
- Width (at hilum): variable (range: 6.0–12.0 cm)
- Depth (AP): <6.0 cm (range 3.0–8.0 cm)
- Volume Index (adult): 8–34 SVI = Length × Height × Thickness/27

Note: the depth measurement may be done in either the longitudinal or transverse axis images; if the coronal plane is used for the longitudinal axis of the spleen, the depth cannot be measured in the same image.

Spleen

Sonographic Finding(s)	Clinical Presentation	Differential Diagnosis	Next Step

Inferior border of spleen extends past mid left kidney or the spleen appears extremely prominent
Echogenicity may be normal or decreased
	Associated with one or more of the following:
	Heart failure
	Portal hypertension
	Leukemia
	Lymphoma
	Hepatitis
	Mononucleosis
	Infectious processes
	Hemolytic anemias
	Also may be seen with:
	   Glycogen storage disease
	   Malaria
	   Myelofibrosis
		Splenomegaly	The underlying cause of splenomegaly cannot always be determined from ultrasound exam

Anechoic to echogenic "mass" or collection within spleen, between splenic parenchyma and capsule, or adjacent to spleen Acoustic enhancement possible	Trauma Labs: decreased hematocrit with significant hemorrhage	Hematoma types: Parenchymal Subcapsular Perisplenic	Document evidence of rupture (fluid) or hematoma formation Follow-up for development of splenosis (implantation of ectopic splenic tissue on intraperitoneal surfaces)
"Mass" with irregular borders with/without septa or complex internal echoes (fluid collection) Hypoechoic mass Splenomegaly Artifact from air within mass	LUQ pain Pleural pain Fever Septicemia Labs: elevated WBC, bacteremia	Abscess Hematoma	Left plural fluid collection may be present
Target lesion(s) or Bull's-eye lesion(s) Splenomegaly	Immunosuppressed patient Labs: positive for candidiasis	Fungal abscess	

continued

Spleen—*cont'd*

Sonographic Finding(s)	Clinical Presentation	Differential Diagnosis	Next Step
Small "mass(es)" noted near splenic hilum or adjacent to spleen; echotexture resembles spleen tissue	Asymptomatic	Accessory spleen(s) Lymphadenopathy	May mimic: pancreas disease, pathology of left adrenal gland or upper pole of left kidney
Unable to locate spleen in LUQ	Patient denies history of splenectomy	Asplenia Ectopic spleen	Normal spleen may be too small or too superior to locate with sonography
Anechoic circular structure within spleen	Asymptomatic History of trauma, pancreatic pseudocyst or hydatid disease	Cyst(s) Resolved infarct Lymphangioma (multiple cysts) Pancreatic pseudocyst	Uncommon finding; majority are associated with nonparasitic cause
Echogenic foci scattered throughout spleen	History of infectious disease	Granulomatous disease Tuberculosis	Echogenicities may represent arterial calcifications

Hyperechoic homogenous "mass(es)"	Asymptomatic	Hemangioma	Hemangiomas in the spleen may have a more varied appearance than those found in the liver
Wedge-shaped hypoechoic defect more commonly noted at border Coarse echotexture	History of vascular disease (embolus or thrombosis)	Infarction	Multiple lesions may be present Infarcts will progress to calcification
Focal hypoechoic mass Large, heterogenous mass	Asymptomatic *or* History of lymphoma or other primary cancer	Lymphoma Leukemia Metastases	Liver and kidneys may be involved in any of the disease processes
Target lesions	History of melanoma, breast, colon, or lung cancer	Metastases (uncommon) Fungal abscess	

Patient Preparation

- No preparation is required, although if included in a complete abdomen examination, the patient may be fasting.

Equipment and Technical Factors

- A curved linear multihertz transducer is commonly used; a sector/vector transducer may be needed for intercostal imaging.
- Color Doppler imaging may be used to distinguish between vascular and nonvascular structures.

Imaging Protocol

- Longitudinal axis images through the medial, mid, and lateral aspects of each kidney are obtained; if scanning the coronal plane for the left kidney, then the anterior, mid, and inferior aspects must be documented. Echogenicity should be compared with that of the liver and spleen.

- Transverse axis images should be obtained through the superior, mid, and inferior aspects of each kidney; the transverse lateral scan plane may be used to obtain these images of the left kidney.
- A variety of transducer placements (scan planes) may be used to obtain diagnostic images of the kidneys; therefore, each image must be labeled accurately to avoid confusion. A coronal scan plane provides a longitudinal and width image of the kidney.
- A variety of patient positions may be used: supine, decubitus, oblique, prone, or upright.
- Longitudinal and transverse axis images of the urinary bladder should be included in the examination; color Doppler imaging may be used to document the urine jets. The female urethra may be evaluated with transperineal imaging.

Variants

- Dromedary hump, hypertrophic column of Bertin, and extrarenal pelvis may be seen; the size of kidneys may vary with age, body habitus, sex, and state of hydration.

Sonographic Measurements

Kidneys

- Length: 9.0–13.0 cm
- Width (at hilum): 5.0 cm
- Depth (AP): 5.0–7.0 cm
- Volume: $(L \times W \times D) \times 0.49$

- Renal sinus thickness may be measured: one half the thickness (depth, AP) of the kidney.
- Cortical thickness may be measured from the base of the pyramid to the renal capsule (approximately 1.0 cm is normal) or by subtracting the renal sinus thickness from the total kidney thickness.

Urinary bladder

- Prevoid and postvoid volume measurements may be done and a residual volume calculated; distended bladder wall measures 3.0–6.0 cm.

Urinary System

Sonographic Finding(s)	Clinical Presentation	Differential Diagnosis	Next Step
Normal to small kidney(s) with very large renal sinus Cortical thinning; cortical thickness <1.0 cm	Asymptomatic	Normal aging process Sinus lipomatosis	
Single/multiple cysts in renal cortex Size is variable; may be very large Closely spaced cysts may appear as one large cyst with septations ("kissing cysts")	Asymptomatic History of long-term dialysis	Development of cysts related to aging ACKD Resolved hematoma Multicystic dysplastic kidney (child) Tuberous sclerosis	"Cyst" that connects with collecting system may indicate hydronephrosis May require a renal Doppler study to demonstrate amount of viable parenchyma remaining

Complex cystic structure arising from renal cortex (septated, internal echoes, possible calcifications) No flow with color Doppler imaging	Asymptomatic *or* Possible flank pain Hematuria Fever Chills Labs: WBC in urine; hematuria	Atypical cortical cyst Hemorrhagic cyst Infected cyst Abscess Tumor Prominent vessel Aneurysm Hematoma	Pus or blood clot may be present in the urinary bladder
Normal kidney with small, hyperechoic structure in cortex	Asymptomatic *or* Painless or painful hematuria (hemorrhage) Hypertension Labs: blood in urine	Angiomyolipoma (more common in females aged 40–60 years) Small RCC (incidental finding)	Power Doppler may be useful to distinguish from RCC Blood clot may be present in urinary bladder

continued

Urinary System—*cont'd*

Sonographic Finding(s)	Clinical Presentation	Differential Diagnosis	Next Step

Hypoechoic to echogenic mass in renal cortex
Variable size
Large mass distorts renal shape
	Asymptomatic
	or
	Possible:
	  Hematuria
	  Hypertension
	  Weight loss
	  Palpable mass
	  Anemia
	  Dysuria
	Patient on immunosuppressants or diabetic
	Labs: elevated BUN, creatinine, WBC
		RCC
		Adenoma
		Angiomyolipoma (hamartoma)
		Abscess
		Fungal infection
			Liver, contralateral kidney, IVC, renal veins, and lymph nodes may demonstrate metastases
			RCC tumor extension or thrombus may be found in IVC
			Abnormal LFT if liver metastases are present

Normal kidney with cystic structure noted at renal hilum Connects with calyces in transverse view	Asymptomatic	Extrarenal pelvis Aneurysm Dilated proximal ureter	Lack of connection with renal pelvis contradicts diagnosis of hydronephrosis Finding collapses when patient is prone Can mimic parapelvic cyst, hydronephrosis, or calyceal diverticula
Cystic structure noted adjacent to renal pelvis May displace renal pelvis and calyces but does not communicate with renal pelvis May mimic hydronephrosis or demonstrate concurrent hydronephrosis	Asymptomatic *or* Possible fever Labs: elevated BUN, creatinine (if obstructed), bacteriuria, leukocytosis	Parapelvic cyst Extrarenal pelvis Lymph node Abscess Hematoma Anechoic lymphoma	If patient is symptomatic or lymphoma is suspected, evaluate lymph nodes and urinary bladder for presence of disease Extrarenal pelvis will collapse when patient is prone

continued

Urinary System—*cont'd*

Sonographic Finding(s)	Clinical Presentation	Differential Diagnosis	Next Step
Large kidneys with multiple irregular cysts Loss of reniform shape Remainder of kidney possibly echogenic Decreased/no visualization of renal sinus	Flank pain Dysuria Hematuria Oliguria Hypertension Palpable flank masses Labs: elevated BUN, creatinine	ADPKD ACKD	Associated with liver and pancreatic cystic disease
Normal kidney; echogenic focus with shadowing noted in renal sinus May be multiple	Hematuria Flank pain Fever Chills Nausea Vomiting Dysuria Renal colic Hematuria	Renal calculus (nephrolithiasis)	Clot or calculus may be present in the urinary bladder Use color Doppler imaging to demonstrate "twinkle" artifact Not all echogenic foci in a kidney are stones!

	Hereditary More common in males Labs: bacteriuria, blood in urine		
Normal to enlarged kidney with dilated renal pelvis with/without dilated ureter May see cortical thinning (cortical thickness <1.0 cm)	Asymptomatic *or* Back/flank pain Renal colic Hematuria Pregnancy History of renal calculi Use of diuretics	Hydronephrosis Pseudo or transient hydronephrosis Reflux	Clot or calculus may be present in the urinary bladder Cortical thickness grading: 1 mild 2 moderate—no cortical thinning 3 severe—cortical thinning
Normal to large kidney(s) with dilated renal pelvis and echoes within pelvis Possible renal stones	Fever Chills Flank pain UTI Labs: bacteremia, pyuria	Pyonephrosis Complication of hydronephrosis	Associated with staghorn calculi (radiograph needed to confirm) and stagnant urine Urinary bladder condition may be present *continued*

Urinary System—*cont'd*

Sonographic Finding(s)	Clinical Presentation	Differential Diagnosis	Next Step
Dilated tubular structure(s) noted in the retroperitoneum with/without hydronephrosis No flow with color Doppler imaging	Pain (associated with hydronephrosis) Labs: increased BUN, creatinine	Hydroureter Dilated vessel or bowel loop	Demonstrate the ureter to termination
Small to nonexistent kidney (little or no parenchyma) with massive renal pelvis Cortical thickness <1.0 cm With/without dilated ureter	Asymptomatic *or* Flank pain Infection Nausea Vomiting Dysuria Fever Chills	Long-standing severe hydronephrosis from ureteral calculi, tumor or UPJ stricture	Evaluate bladder for presence of clot or calculus

	Labs: elevated BUN, creatinine, microscopic hematuria, azotemia/uremia		
Large, hypoechoic kidneys with decreased or no visualization of renal sinus	Nausea Vomiting Pain Dysuria Polyuria Anuria Hypertension Hematuria Labs: elevated BUN, creatinine, WBC	Acute infection Diffuse lymphoma	Lymphoma may be present in the urinary bladder Renal lymphoma is more common in patients with non-Hodgkin's lymphoma
Large, normal to echogenic kidneys with decreased or no visualization of renal sinus	Oliguria Recent fever/sore throat Hematuria	Acute glomerulonephritis	Document distention/size of urinary bladder

continued

Urinary System—*cont'd*

Sonographic Finding(s)	Clinical Presentation	Differential Diagnosis	Next Step
Renal pyramids well seen (prominent)	Fatigue Nausea Peripheral edema Joint pain Proteinuria Labs: elevated BUN, creatinine, WBC; decreased GFR		
Normal-sized kidney(s) with enlargement of corticomedullary area and decreased echogenicity and loss of definition Possible overall enlarged kidneys OR focal involvement (may appear as "mass") Possible mild hydronephrosis	Asymptomatic *or* Weight loss Recurrent UTI Urinary frequency Labs: elevated BUN, creatinine, WBC; bacteriuria	Acute pyelonephritis Focal presentation also known as acute lobar nephronia or acute focal bacterial nephritis Lymphoma RCC Abscess	Associated with diabetes, urinary obstruction, pregnancy, urinary reflux, immunosuppression, or known renal lesion Color Doppler imaging may be useful to demonstrate hyperemia in area(s) of acute infection

			Evidence of tumor or thrombus in renal vein, IVC, or bladder related to RCC or lymphoma
Large, hypoechoic kidneys with decreased or no visualization of renal sinus Marked increase in AP diameter Renal pyramids may be hypoechoic and large OR hyperechoic	Nausea Vomiting Edema Oliguria Hematuria Hypotension Muscle necrosis Flank pain Infection Sepsis Labs: elevated BUN, creatinine, WBC	ATN as a result of ischemic event or toxic insult Nephrocalcinosis	ATN may be associated with development of papillary necrosis, which causes nephrocalcinosis

continued

Urinary System—*cont'd*

Sonographic Finding(s)	Clinical Presentation	Differential Diagnosis	Next Step

Small, echogenic kidney(s)
Parenchymal scarring may be noted (irregular contour of kidney)
Cortical thinning; cortical thickness <1.0 cm
	Malaise/fatigue
	Anorexia
	Hypotension
	Oliguria
	Anemia
	Repeated UTIs
	Possible:
	  Fever
	  Nausea/vomiting
	  Flank pain
	  Dysuria
	  Hypertension
	Labs: elevated BUN, creatinine; decreasing GFR
		Chronic renal failure
		Chronic pyelonephritis (scarring)
		Normal atrophy of aging
			Associated with numerous underlying renal disease processes
			Urinary bladder should be noted if finding related to normal aging process

Normal-sized kidney(s) with focal area(s) of decreased echogenicity	Nausea Vomiting Weight loss Anorexia Fatigue Pain Hematuria	Focal lymphoma Cyst(s) RCC Focal pyelonephritis	Renal involvement more common in patients with non-Hodgkin's lymphoma
Normal kidney echogenicity with hyperechoic pyramids with/without shadowing	Asymptomatic *or* Hematuria Flank pain Fever Dysuria Labs: microscopic hematuria, pyuria	Nephrocalcinosis Medullary sponge kidney ATN	In symptomatic patients, evaluate urinary bladder for presence of bilateral urine jets (patent ureters)

continued

Urinary System—*cont'd*

Sonographic Finding(s)	Clinical Presentation	Differential Diagnosis	Next Step
Multiple renal calculi and dilated calyces	Renal colic (flank pain) Dysuria Hematuria Pyuria Labs: Hematuria, bacteremia, low urine specific gravity; elevated BUN, creatinine with obstruction	Papillary necrosis	Associated with ATN
Solid mass in renal sinus, ureter or bladder Isoechoic to hypoechoic Hydronephrosis may be noted Enlarged lymph nodes may be noted	Painless hematuria Gross hematuria Blood clots in urine Possible fever and flank pain Labs: elevated BUN, creatinine (obstruction), WBC, bacteriuria	TCC (more common in men) SCC (associated with chronic infection, irritation, kidney stones, drug use)	Tumor or blood clots may be present in urinary bladder Metastatic spread to contralateral kidney and lymph nodes or tumor extension into renal vein(s) and IVC

Kidney has a "lumpy" appearance	Asymptomatic	Fetal lobulation	Normal feature of kidney development in utero that may persist into adulthood
Unable to locate kidney in renal fossa	Asymptomatic Patient denies surgical removal of kidney	Ectopic kidney Unilateral renal agenesis	Evaluate pelvis to locate kidney Ectopic kidney in pelvis may demonstrate malrotation
Unable to identify inferior poles of kidneys, poles seem to lie more medially and posterior than normal; slight malrotation may be noted Connection of solid tissue between inferior poles of the kidneys anterior to great vessels	Asymptomatic *or* History of UTI	Horseshoe kidneys	Accurate length measurement of kidneys may not be possible Associated with reproductive system anomalies

continued

Urinary System—cont'd

Sonographic Finding(s)	Clinical Presentation	Differential Diagnosis	Next Step
Both kidneys located on same side of abdomen; superior pole of one kidney attached to inferior pole of contralateral kidney One or both kidneys may be malrotated Hydronephrosis of one or both kidneys	Asymptomatic or History of UTI	Fused renal ectopia (also known as "crossed fused renal ectopia")	Measurements of kidneys may not be possible because of fusion and malrotation Associated with reproductive tract anomalies Evaluate bladder for urine jets at normal location
Triangular echogenic focus noted between the mid and upper sections of the kidney	Asymptomatic	Junctional parenchymal defect	May also be seen with an interventricular septum Remnant of fetal renal lobes

Parenchymal tissue separates two areas of the echogenic renal sinus Kidney may be normal or somewhat larger in size May be noted bilaterally	Asymptomatic	Bifid renal pelvis Duplex collecting system	Mildest form of kidney duplication Renal pelvis is singular at the renal hilum
Duplication of the renal collecting system with duplication of ureters Ureters may rejoin distal to kidney and proximal to bladder Kidney is usually larger than normal May be bilateral	Asymptomatic History of urinary reflux and pyelonephritis	Duplex collecting system: Partial Complete	Reproductive anomalies may be present

continued

Urinary System—*cont'd*

Sonographic Finding(s)	Clinical Presentation	Differential Diagnosis	Next Step

Small kidney with decreased cortical thickness
Narrowing of vessel; calcifications may be noted
Direct evaluation of the renal artery:
PSV in renal artery >180 cm/s
RAR >3.5
Indirect evaluation or renal flow:
  Acceleration time >0.1
  Acceleration index <3.78
Loss of early systolic peak
  Tardus parvus waveform
  RI > 0.7
  Intrarenal artery S/D ratio <0.23
	Asymptomatic
	or
	Hypertension
	CHF
	Renal failure
		Renal artery stenosis	Associated with:
			  Atherosclerosis
			  Fibromuscular dysplasia
			  Arteritis
			  Renal artery aneurysm
			  Irradiation
			  Emboli
			  Thrombosis
			  Hematoma
			  Neoplasm
			Indirect method requires sampling several areas of kidney
			Direct evaluation may be difficult because of multiple renal arteries, bowel gas, or patient body habitus

Cyst in bladder near trigone area Hydroureter may be noted Bladder wall may be thickened	Asymptomatic *or* History of bladder infection, renal duplication	Ureterocele	Associated with ureteral duplication or may be an isolated finding Demonstrate urine jets with color Doppler imaging
Echogenic mass/structure within bladder	Asymptomatic Labs: blood in urine; elevated BUN, creatinine (obstruction)	Catheter Foreign body Calculi Tumor Fungus ball Blood clot Polyp	Demonstrate mobility of mass/structure
Solid mass projecting into bladder lumen	Painless hematuria	Bladder tumor Papilloma TCC SCC	Most common cause TCC Metastases from kidneys, uterus, cervix, prostate, rectum *continued*

Urinary System—*cont'd*

Sonographic Finding(s)	Clinical Presentation	Differential Diagnosis	Next Step
		Metastatic Cystitis Benign prostatic hypertrophy Blood clots Endometriosis	

Bladder wall appears thick
  when bladder is distended
May be diffuse or focal
	Frequency
	Dysuria
	Lower abdominal pain
	Nocturia
	Hematuria
	Diabetes
	History of schistosomiasis
	  infection
	Labs: bacteriuria, blood in
	  urine
		Chronic cystitis
		Neurogenic bladder
		Focal bladder mass
		  (TCC)
			Echoes or fluid/fluid level
			  in bladder related to
			  hemorrhage
			Adherent blood clot
			Air in bladder wall associated
			  with emphysematous cystitis
			  (diabetics)
			Schistosomiasis infection may
			  lead to development of SCC

Bladder wall has "ruffled" appearance from multiple outpouchings Variable in size (can be as large as the bladder); decrease in size when bladder is emptied	Asymptomatic *or* History of UTI Labs: elevated BUN, creatinine if obstruction is extensive	Bladder diverticuli Hydroureter	Associated with urine stasis and infection Seen with cystitis, congenital defects, or bladder obstruction

Patient Preparation

- Fasting for 6 to 8 hours before the scan is preferable, but it may be done without preparation.

Equipment and Technical Factors

- A curved linear is the most common transducer used; a sector/vector transducer improves access through small acoustic windows.

Imaging Protocol

Minimum documentation images for the area of interest

- Longitudinal and transverse axes images should be obtained of the area of interest.
- The abdominal aorta and IVC proximal, mid, and distal portions should be documented in longitudinal and transverse images; vessel branches and tributaries should be included at the documentation levels.
- Measurements are performed as required by protocol or presence of pathology.

- Measurements must be performed according to the plane (perpendicular to the longitudinal axis) of the vessel because of angulation or tortuosity that occurs with enlargement or aging.
- To avoid confusion from the variety transducer placements that may be used to obtain diagnostic images of the area of interest, each image must be labeled accurately for scan plane and anatomy demonstrated.
- Images of healthy adrenal glands in the adult may be difficult to obtain.

Sonographic Measurements

There are no specific measurements for peritoneal and retroperitoneal cavities with or without the presence of disease.

Aorta

Outer to outer diameter: upper limits of normal

- 2.5–3.0 cm at the diaphragm
- 2.0 cm at midabdomen

- 1.8–1.0 cm at the bifurcation
- Ectasia: abdominal aortic enlargement <3.0 cm
- Aneurysm: focal dilatation of abdominal aorta >3.0 cm

IVC

- Less than 2.5 cm to a maximum of 4.0 cm; varies with respiration

Adult adrenal gland

- 3.0–5.0 cm length
- 2.0–3.0 cm width
- 3.0–6.0 mm depth (thickness)

Abdomen and Retroperitoneum

Sonographic Finding(s)	Clinical Presentation	Differential Diagnosis	Next Step
Aorta is enlarged but is <3.0 cm in diameter (perpendicular to longitudinal axis of vessel, outer to outer wall) Aorta may demonstrate angulation or tortuosity	Asymptomatic Elderly patient	Ectasia of the aorta	Ensure accurate measurement technique for follow-up studies May slowly progress to AAA
Aorta is enlarged, >3.0 cm in diameter (perpendicular to longitudinal axis of vessel, outer to outer wall)	Asymptomatic Pulsatile abdominal mass Abdominal bruit	AAA (fusiform)	5.0–6.0 cm diameter: likely surgical intervention ≥7.0 cm: high risk of rupture and surgical intervention

Aorta is dilated circumferentially but may bulge somewhat toward patient's left Homogenous clot may be noted along anterior/anterolateral wall Aorta may demonstrate angulation or tortuosity Color Doppler demonstrates turbulent, swirling flow			Demonstrate relationship of AAA to renal arteries or extension into common iliac arteries Lumen may be measured
Pulsating or moving "flap" within aorta or aneurysm Color Doppler imaging demonstrates blood flow on both sides of the "flap"	History of AAA Severe chest and back pain	Dissecting aorta (dissecting aneurysm) Originates in thoracic aorta and extends into abdominal aorta	Life-threatening finding Demonstrate extent of dissection and relationship to renal arteries

continued

Abdomen and Retroperitoneum—cont'd

Sonographic Finding(s)	Clinical Presentation	Differential Diagnosis	Next Step

Aorta appears to have internal linear bright echogenicities *or* appears as two tubes, one with bright walls
 	
Fluid may be noted around aorta
	Surgical intervention for AAA	Aortic graft
		  End to end
		  Endoluminal
			Fluid collection is a common postsurgical finding
			Brightness of graft walls from type of graft material
			Graft should be followed for patency, development of aneurysm or pseudoaneurysm at anastomosis sites, infection, leakage, and degeneration of graft

IVC is compressed, dilated, or deviated from normal lie	Symptoms associated with underlying disease process	IVC dilation	Related to effects of cardiac disease (dilated IVC), hepatomegaly

Intraluminal homogenous mass with/without obstruction of IVC Color Doppler imaging demonstrates flow around mass or obstruction of IVC	Symptoms increase with degree of obstruction: Leg edema Low back/pelvic pain GI complaints Labs: abnormal liver or renal values	IVC thrombosis	Associated with extension of lower extremity or pelvic venous thrombus, clot from tumor invasion, or Budd-Chiari syndrome Complete thrombosis is life threatening
Intraluminal nodules/mass within IVC with/without obstruction	Symptoms and lab values associated with underlying disease process	IVC tumor	Associated with direct or venous extension of RCC or HCC, primary tumor of IVC (rare) *continued*

Abdomen and Retroperitoneum—*cont'd*

Sonographic Finding(s)	Clinical Presentation	Differential Diagnosis	Next Step
Color Doppler imaging demonstrates blood flow within and around nodule/ mass			
Multiple hypoechoic masses, may be indistinct or matted, surrounding aorta, SMA, IVC, celiac Aorta may be "lifted" off of spine SMA appears "sandwiched"; celiac trunk and SMA may be straightened May be noted at liver, kidney and splenic hila	Asymptomatic Vague complaints Possible weight loss May have abnormal lab values for liver and kidney function if either are the primary cause	Lymphadenopathy Spread of infection or malignancy	Liver, kidney, remainder of retroperitoneum, and spleen disease may be present

Appearance of a "kidney" in the abdomen (pseudokidney sign) Mass with central hyperechoic area and surrounding hypoechoic layer Does not compress with transducer pressure	Asymptomatic, incidental finding May have bowel complaints May have pain at site	Carcinoma Lymphoma Chronic: Crohn's disease	Evaluate for lymph node involvement, liver and spleen disease
Anechoic fluid surrounds abdominal organs (no fluid in bare area of liver); bowel loops free floating within fluid	History of carcinoma, cirrhosis of liver	Ascites	Document amount and location(s) of fluid Evaluate liver, ovaries for presence of disease

continued

Abdomen and Retroperitoneum—*cont'd*

Sonographic Finding(s)	Clinical Presentation	Differential Diagnosis	Next Step
Abdominal hypoechoic fluid; bowel loops matted and not moving with respiration	History of carcinoma, infection	Infected fluid Fluid containing metastases	Document amount and location(s) of fluid Evaluate liver, ovaries for presence of disease

Solid mass superior to kidney
May displace vessels, kidney
	Hypertension
	Possible incidental finding
	Labs: excessive androgens, estrogens, aldosterone, glucocorticoids, epinephrine, or norepinephrine
		Adrenal tumor
		Adult:
		  Adenoma
		  Malignancy
		  Metastases
		  Metastases from lung, breast, colon, stomach, or kidney
		Pheochromocytoma
		Child: Neuroblastoma
			Document that mass is nonrenal
			Color Doppler imaging may be used to document displacement of vessels
			Metastatic spread to IVC, lymph nodes and diaphragm may be present

Cystic structure superior/ anterior to kidney; may contain echoes May have calcification	Asymptomatic Hypertension Possible pain if hemorrhage	Adrenal cyst (more common in female patients) Pheochromocytoma	Demonstrate that cyst is nonrenal
Hydroureter(s) without evidence of calculi or external mass causing obstruction	Symptoms associated with hydronephrosis Labs: elevated BUN, creatinine if hydronephrosis is present	Retroperitoneal fibrosis	May be related to metastases or aneurysm Evaluate liver for presence of disease
Fluid collection adjacent to kidney(s) or in retroperitoneum	Pain Fever Chills	Urinoma Hemorrhage Abscess	Evaluate kidney for rupture (urinoma or hemorrhage)

continued

Abdomen and Retroperitoneum—*cont'd*

Sonographic Finding(s)	Clinical Presentation	Differential Diagnosis	Next Step
Grey Turner's sign may be noted (discoloration of flanks from blood in retroperitoneum)	Trauma Surgery Chronic urinary obstruction (urinoma) Labs: elevated WBC with abscess; decreased hematocrit with hemorrhage		Chronic hydronephrosis may lead to development of urinoma Hemorrhage may be related to AAA rupture
Fluid posterior to stomach (lesser sac)	History of pancreatitis Labs: elevated amylase, lipase, WBC	Pancreatic fluid Massive ascites	Pancreatic pseudocyst may be present Massive ascites may force fluid through the epiploic foramen into lesser sac
Complex fluid collection/ "mass" in abdominal wall	History of trauma, surgery Anticoagulant therapy	Rectus sheath hematoma	Ensure that the "mass" is not part of the abdominal cavity

Follows tissue planes (oval rather than round) Anechoic to echogenic "mass" May demonstrate echogenicities with some acoustic shadowing	Labs: decreased hematocrit; elevated WBC	Abscess	by having the patient breathe while high-frequency linear array transducer is maintained in place over area of interest Abscess may occur at site of incision; scan by using a sterile technique

Patient Preparation

- Fasting for 6 to 8 hours before the examination(s) is preferable, but it may be accomplished without preparation.

Equipment and Technical Factors

- A curved linear or linear array (thin patient) is the transducer of choice.

Imaging Protocol

- Longitudinal and transverse axes images should be the area of interest
- To avoid confusion as a result of the variety transducer placements that may be used to obtain diagnostic images of

the area of interest, each image must be labeled accurately for scan plane and anatomy demonstrated.

- Normal bowel should demonstrate peristalsis and movement of fluid through the lumen.
- The graded compression technique is used to differentiate normal versus abnormal bowel.

Sonographic Measurements

- Bowel diameter: <5.0 mm
- Appendix: <6.0 mm in diameter, <2.0 mm in wall thickness

Bowel

Sonographic Finding(s)	Clinical Presentation	Differential Diagnosis	Next Step
Appearance of a "kidney" in the abdomen (pseudokidney sign) "Mass" with hyperechoic center with surrounding hypoechoic layer (target sign) "Mass" does not compress with transducer pressure Decreased peristalsis may be noted	Asymptomatic May have bowel complaints: Cramping Nausea Vomiting Weight loss May have pain at site Anemia and palpable mass associated with lymphoma	Carcinoma Lymphoma Crohn's disease	Associated with history of ulcerative colitis
Prominent appendix noted at terminal ileum/cecum Increased diameter and wall thickening	Severe periumbilical to right lower quadrant pain Fever	Acute appendicitis Bowel tumor Typhlitis (cecitis)	Evaluate point of pain as indicated by patient

continued

Bowel—*cont'd*

Sonographic Finding(s)	Clinical Presentation	Differential Diagnosis	Next Step
Noncompressible Positive McBurney's sign (pain with release of pressure at McBurney's point) With/without fluid within or adjacent to appendix With/without appendicolith	Chills Nausea Vomiting Labs: elevated WBC		Female patient: evaluate pelvis for ectopic pregnancy or rupture ovarian cyst Evaluate right kidney for retroperitoneal fluid collection Possible abscess or rupture
Complex mass in RLQ Calculi or air may be noted within the mass Free fluid may be noted near cecum	Fever Chills Pain History of appendectomy Labs: elevated WBC	Appendiceal abscess Bowel mass In a female patient consider ovarian mass or PID	Complication of appendicitis or appendectomy
Thickened wall in small or large bowel; matted bowel loops	Diarrhea (possibly bloody) Lower abdominal pain Cramps	Inflammatory bowel disease: Crohn's disease	Evaluate sites of pain, remainder of bowel, especially the appendix

May mimic neoplasm	Fever Weight loss Attacks precipitated by stress	Ulcerative colitis (increased risk of carcinoma)	May mimic appendicitis
Multiple fluid-filled loops of bowel Little or no peristalsis; to and fro sloshing of fluid within bowel	Abdominal pain Vomiting Constipation Weight loss	Paralytic ileus	Associated with obstructed bowel, mass, intussusception, hernia. lymphoma, adhesions, SMA syndrome
Thickened bowel wall Echogenic areas adjacent to bowel Increased echogenicity around bowel (thyroid in the abdomen sign)	Pain Fever Chills History of diverticulosis: Cramping Lower abdominal pain Constipation Distention	Diverticulitis	Associated with abscess, development of sinus tracts, and peritonitis

SUPERFICIAL STRUCTURES

Patient Preparation

- No preparation is required.

Equipment and Technical Factors

- A high-frequency linear array is used for imaging the breast.
- To examine large superficial structure pathology, use a curved linear transducer to place the anatomy into the widest portion of the image.

Imaging Protocol

- Longitudinal and transverse axes images of the organ or area of interest
- When the breast is imaged, standardized labeling must be used (quadrant, radial/antiradial, clock face and distance from nipple).
- Correlate with mammography findings: for example, Bi-Rads classification and location.

Patient positioning

- Supine with ipsilateral arm raised or slightly oblique with ipsilateral arm raised (helpful for scanning left breast or large breast)
- For a small-breasted patient, supine with arm down reduces compression of the breast tissue from tightened skin.
- Light transducer pressure is used to avoid compression of tissues and structures; compression is used in the evaluation of suspicious areas or masses.

Variants

- Tail of Spence, ectopic breast tissue, accessory (supernumerary) nipples.

Sonographic Measurements

- Length, depth, and width of the cyst, mass, or other diseased area.

Breast

Sonographic Finding(s)	Clinical Presentation	Differential Diagnosis	Next Step
Solid breast mass, homogenous with low level echoes, with/without acoustic attenuation Oval: "broader than tall"; compressible Well defined with smooth margins; gentle lobulations may be noted Calcifications may be noted	Palpable breast lump Nontender, firm, rubbery Pregnant patient may have noted rapid enlargement (from hormonal stimulation) Highly suspicious in postmenopausal women	Fibroadenoma	Color Doppler imaging and vocal fremitus may aid in benign determination to demonstrate peripheral flow around mass Demonstrate disruption or invasion of tissue planes Correlate with Bi-Rads classification
Hyperechoic parenchyma with/without sound attenuation and shadowing; may present as hyperechoic mass Cysts or cyst clusters may be noted Ductal ectasia may be noted	Cyclic pattern of breast discomfort or pain, especially before menses Increase in breast firmness Lumpy breast Possible nipple discharge	Fibrocystic change	Benign condition but family history of breast cancer increases risk in presence of ductal ectasia

continued

Breast—*cont'd*

Sonographic Finding(s)	Clinical Presentation	Differential Diagnosis	Next Step
Round/oval cystic structure(s) Septations may be noted Low-level echoes may be noted	Palpable to nonpalpable mass May note change in size with menstrual cycle May have pain on palpation Highly suspicious in postmenopausal women	Cyst(s) Galactocele Hemorrhagic cyst Hematoma Mastitis	Evaluate internal echoes within cyst; advances in technology reveal many previously anechoic cysts to have internal echoes; compare with previous sonogram Aspiration may be needed to confirm as benign Correlate with Bi-Rads classification
Oval, hypoechoic structure with echogenic central area Noted in axilla or possibly intramammary	Possible palpable mass Mammographic finding	Prominent lymph node	Evaluate same area in contralateral breast for similar finding Color Doppler imaging may be used to demonstrate vessels in hilum

Hypoechoic solid mass of variable shape; some attenuation Irregular margins/speculated Invasion or disruption of tissue planes Microlobulations "Taller than broad" Not compressible Ductal extension	If palpable: painless, hard and fixed in position Skin changes may be noted Receding nipple or discharge from nipple Microcalcifications on mammogram	Infiltrating ductal carcinoma (most common) Infiltrating lobular carcinoma Mucinous carcinoma Tubular carcinoma Papillary carcinoma	Color Doppler imaging and fremitus may be used to confirm finding Evaluate entire breast for multifocal disease (as requested) Evaluate axillary region for enlarged lymph nodes Correlate with Bi-Rads classification
Prominent tubular structure(s) Possible stellate pattern	Pregnant or lactating woman Nonpregnant or lactating woman	Ductal ectasia	In nonpregnant or lactating woman, evaluate for cause of prominent duct; possible papilloma of duct

continued

Breast—*cont'd*

Sonographic Finding(s)	Clinical Presentation	Differential Diagnosis	Next Step
Ill-defined solid-appearing mass with irregular walls with/ without posterior enhancement May have variable appearance depending on stage of inflammation	History of mastitis Skin erythema Swelling Pain Fever	Abscess	In a patient without history of mastitis, consider evaluation for inflammatory carcinoma
Diffuse skin thickening with increase in echogenicity of subcutaneous fat Disruption of tissue planes Thickened Cooper's ligaments Color Doppler imaging demonstrates hypervascularity of tissues Dilated superficial veins may be noted	Skin erythema, edema, and thickening "Orange peel" appearance of skin Flattening and retraction of nipple Swollen, painful, hard breast	Inflammatory carcinoma Mastitis	Highly invasive and aggressive type of cancer Bilateral disease is possible Biopsy needed to differentiate from mastitis

Closely spaced lines within implant	Asymptomatic	Normal augmented breast	Injection port may be noted in shell of implant
Echogenic lines within the implant (stepladder sign)	Asymptomatic Change in appearance/consistency of breast	Intracapsular silicone implant rupture	Evaluate for evidence of extracapsular rupture
Echogenicity with "snowstorm" appearance external to implant May demonstrate a "dirty" shadow	Change in appearance or consistency of breast Tenderness or burning sensation Breast lump/mass	Extracapsular silicone implant rupture	Document presence of silicone granuloma

Patient Preparation

- No preparation is required for neck and thyroid imaging.

Equipment and Technical Factors

- A high-frequency linear array is used for imaging the neck and thyroid.
- To image large superficial structure pathology, a curved linear or sector transducer with a stand-off pad to place the anatomy into the wider portion of the image may be used.

Imaging Protocol

- Longitudinal and transverse axes images of the organ or area of interest with the neck slightly extended (hyperextension is contraindicated).
- Demonstrate relational anatomy.

Variants

- Pyramidal lobe of the thyroid

Sonographic Measurements

Thyroid

- Length: 4.0–6.0 cm
- Width: 1.3–1.8 cm
- Depth (AP): 1.3–1.8 cm
- Isthmus: 3.0 mm

Neck

- Length, depth, and width of cyst, mass, or diseased area.

Neck and Thyroid

Sonographic Finding(s)	Clinical Presentation	Differential Diagnosis	Next Step
Solid mass(es) more echogenic than thyroid with hypoechoic halo Well defined Possible cystic degeneration or "eggshell" calcification noted Predominately cystic mass(es) May appear complex	Asymptomatic Possible palpable nodule in thyroid	Thyroid adenoma Degenerating adenoma	Adenomas may undergo cystic degeneration and appear as complex mass Do not overlook the isthmus Use light transducer pressure to avoid missing small lesions
Cystic structure with irregular walls and internal echoes	Asymptomatic Possible palpable thyroid nodule	Thyroid cyst (with/without hemorrhage) Degenerating adenoma	Do not overlook the isthmus Use light transducer pressure to avoid missing small lesions *continued*

Neck and Thyroid—*cont'd*

Sonographic Finding(s)	Clinical Presentation	Differential Diagnosis	Next Step
Solitary hypoechoic mass with irregular border and microcalcifications	Asymptomatic	Thyroid carcinoma	Thyroid carcinoma is more common in women
Enlarged lymph node(s) in neck may be noted; the node(s) may be predominately cystic	Palpable hard mass in neck (associated cervical adenopathy)	Papillary	Papillary carcinoma is the most common type
Lesion may be very small to large	Enlarging goiter	Follicular	Anaplastic carcinoma demonstrates rapid growth and is more common in men
Cystic degeneration not usually noted	Pressure symptoms	Medullary	Doppler imaging should be used to evaluate vascularity of mass and node(s)
	Hoarseness	Anaplastic	Biopsy or fine needle aspiration may be needed to determine type of malignancy versus benign
	Cold nodule on nuclear medicine scan		
	Generally a slow growth pattern		
	Labs: abnormal serum calcitonin levels associated with medullary carcinoma		

Sonographic Findings	Clinical Findings	Differential Diagnosis	Notes
Enlarged thyroid with/ without nodules; coarse echotexture May be focal or diffuse asymmetric enlargement	Thyroid enlargement Labs: hypothyroidism	Nontoxic (simple) goiter Thyroiditis Neoplasm	May be related to iodine deficiency or glandular malfunction Goiter is a term that can be used to describe any enlarged thyroid regardless of etiology
Enlarged inhomogeneous thyroid; may be asymmetrically enlarged Focal scarring, ischemia, necrosis, and cyst formation may be noted	Thyroid enlargement Difficulty breathing and swallowing Labs: normal or possible thyrotoxicosis	Toxic multinodular goiter Adenomas	Associated with calcifications
Diffusely enlarged thyroid with decreased echogenicity and hyperemia (increased blood flow) Possible calcifications	Asymptomatic Possibly painful if subacute Hoarseness Labs: possible decreased T3 and T4	Hashimoto's thyroiditis	Most common inflammatory process of thyroid More common in women Color Doppler imaging to demonstrate hyperemia *continued*

Neck and Thyroid—*cont'd*

Sonographic Finding(s)	Clinical Presentation	Differential Diagnosis	Next Step
Diffusely enlarged thyroid with areas of increased and decreased echogenicity	Swelling Pain Fever Palpable thyroid with diffuse or focal enlargement Labs: normal WBC; possible increased T3 and T4	de Quervain thyroiditis/subacute granulomatous thyroiditis	Associated with previous viral infection Color Doppler imaging demonstrates normal or increased blood flow
Enlarged hypoechoic thyroid with hypervascularity May demonstrate as heterogenous	Swelling of neck Labs: elevated T3 and T4	Graves' disease (diffuse toxic goiter or thyrotoxicosis)	Color Doppler imaging demonstrates hypervascularity of gland ("thyroid inferno")

Hypoechoic solid oval-shaped mass found posterior to thyroid and medial to carotid artery Increased vascularity may be noted	History of frequent kidney stones or renal disease Osteopenia Labs: elevated calcium and parathyroid hormone levels	Parathyroid adenoma	Parathyroid glands may be ectopic Mimics posterior thyroid nodule Color Doppler imaging demonstrates increased blood flow in adenoma
Hypoechoic round mass(es) noted near jugular vein May appear as one large mass or several separate masses Areas of cystic degeneration or calcifications may be noted	Palpable mass in neck Pain Fever Skin erythema Labs: increased WBC (inflammatory)	Lymphadenopathy Inflammatory neoplastic	Evaluate both sides of neck for presence of enlarged lymph nodes Document shape of nodes: round nodes are more commonly malignant Malignant nodes may have more heterogenous echotexture and microcalcifications Color Doppler imaging may demonstrate abnormal flow patterns

continued

Neck and Thyroid—*cont'd*

Sonographic Finding(s)	Clinical Presentation	Differential Diagnosis	Next Step
Fluid-filled structure noted lateral and superior to thyroid May have internal echoes	Asymptomatic unless infected	Branchial cleft cyst	Evaluate for presence infection
Fusiform-shaped cyst midline and anterior to trachea	Asymptomatic Palpable mass Sinus tract drainage	Thyroglossal duct cyst	Congenital anomaly Demonstrate that cyst is not within thyroid

PELVIS

Chapter 11 Male Pelvis

Chapter 12 Female Pelvis

Patient Preparation

- Full bladder preparation for the urinary bladder or transabdominal prostate examination.
- Bowel preparation for the transrectal prostate examination.
- No preparation for the scrotal/testicular examination.

Equipment and Technical Factors

A high-frequency linear array is used for imaging the scrotum. Endorectal prostate imaging requires the use of the specialized transrectal transducer. The transrectal transducer should be adequately sheathed for the examination and appropriately disinfected after each use. Published guidelines for disinfection of endocavitary transducers are available. In addition, manufacturer specifications should be followed to avoid damaging the transducer.

Imaging Protocol

- Evaluate and document the longitudinal and transverse axes of the testicle regardless of the position of the testicle within the scrotum.
- Doppler (color, spectral) evaluation and comparison of blood flow in the testes should be documented. Low-flow settings should be used to avoid false-negative findings in cases of suspected torsion. Split-screen method allows flow in both testicles to be compared side by side. Doppler settings are the same for both testicles.
- Evaluate and document the prostate in the transverse axis from the superior aspect (base) to the inferior aspect (apex) and in the longitudinal axis from the midline to each lateral border.

- Evaluate and document the seminal vesicles in the transverse axis of each gland.
- Longitudinal and transverse axes images of the bladder to demonstrate the overall size of the prostate may be done.

Sonographic Measurements

Testicle
- Length: 4.0–5.0 cm
- Width: 2.0–3.0 cm
- Thickness (AP): 2.0–3.0 cm

Prostate
- Length: 2.0–4.0 cm
- Width: 3.9–5.3 cm
- Thickness: 2.1–3.4 cm
- Volume: 13.7 mL
- $V = (\pi/6) \times (L \times W \times T)$

Seminal vesicles
- Length: 2.0–4.0 cm
- Diameter: 1.0 cm

Male Pelvis

Sonographic Finding(s)	Clinical Presentation	Differential Diagnosis	Next Step
Hypoechoic or heterogenous enlarged testicle Possible hydrocele noted Possible that testicular echogenicity and texture are normal Peripheral hyperemia may be noted No or decreased internal testicular flow demonstrated on color Doppler imaging	Scrotal swelling with pain	Testicular torsion	Compare affected testicle appearance with contralateral side Ensure Doppler device is set to normal testicle and not changed for affected testicle Because of peripheral hyperemia, flow may be detected in affected testicle but torsion should not be excluded because of this finding Testicle may demonstrate deceased flow from partial torsion or untwisting at time of exam

Cystic structure noted in epididymis, superior to testicle	Asymptomatic	Spermatocele Epididymal cyst	Evaluate for flow in cystic structure to ensure that the cyst is not a dilated vessel
Fluid surrounds one or both testicles Amount of fluid may be small to massive	Asymptomatic Painful if related to rupture Possible scrotal enlargement if large amount of fluid	Hydrocele Hematocele	Evaluate for echogenicities in fluid that indicate infection or blood (from rupture) Evaluate for other testicular disease, such as infection
Numerous "cysts" or tubular anechoic structures noted near the epididymis; may extend superiorly More common on the left because of drainage of gonadal vein into renal vein Increase in size during Valsalva maneuver	Asymptomatic Problems with fertility Sudden onset may be related to obstruction of venous drainage	Varicocele	Confirm anechoic structures, dilated veins by color Doppler imaging Document vein incompetence during Valsalva maneuver Evaluate pelvis and abdomen for mass or tumor compressing vein (sudden onset)

continued

Pelvis

Male Pelvis—cont'd

Sonographic Finding(s)	Clinical Presentation	Differential Diagnosis	Next Step
Enlarged hypoechoic heterogenous epididymis May demonstrate focal areas of increased echogenicity and calcification Hydrocele may be noted	Acute onset of unilateral scrotal pain Fever, dysuria, malaise History of trauma, UTI, STD, neoplasm, TB, prostatitis Focal tenderness Labs: increased WBC	Epididymitis Chronic epididymitis (hard, palpable mass, injured less painful than acute)	Demonstrate increased blood flow in affected side and compare with contralateral epididymis Compare echogenicity and texture with unaffected side
Decreased echogenicity of testicle; may be focal Scrotal wall thickening may be noted Hyperemia may be noted May develop areas of necrosis	History of epididymitis or viral infection Pain, fever, nausea, and vomiting	Orchitis	Evaluate for concurrent epididymitis Document hyperemia with Doppler imaging
Fluid with echogenicities surrounding testicle	Scrotal pain May be acute or chronic	Pyocele	Evaluate testicle for infection

Wall of scrotum thickened; septations may be present			
Testicle appears atrophied; measures smaller than normal One testicle smaller than the other	History of orchitis	Chronic orchitis	Compare affected testicle with contralateral testicle with 2D and Doppler evaluation
Hypoechoic solid mass in testicle May appear as complex mass Mass may have irregular or smooth borders Calcifications may be present Areas of cystic degeneration may be noted	Asymptomatic enlargement of testicle; palpable mass *or* Enlarged, painful scrotum Possible elevated AFP or hCG	Testicular carcinoma Seminoma Mixed germ cell Nongerm cell Metastases Leukemia Lymphoma	Evaluate both testicles for presence of multiple masses Doppler evaluation of testicles and any masses should be performed Evaluate for metastatic spread to abdomen
"Mass" in scrotum that may contain air and demonstrate peristalsis Movement of mass with Valsalva maneuver	Enlarged scrotum Asymptomatic to painful	Scrotal hernia	Evaluate for peristalsis and blood flow in mass (lack of blood flow may indicate incarceration)

continued

Pelvis

Male Pelvis—cont'd

Sonographic Finding(s)	Clinical Presentation	Differential Diagnosis	Next Step
Enlarged prostate (especially thickness) with variable echogenicity Cystic areas and calcifications may be noted Nodules may be noted Urethra may be displaced posteriorly	Frequency of urination Urgency and feeling of constant fullness Labs: elevated PSA	BPH	Asymmetry of the gland is associated with carcinoma Secondary changes in the bladder may be noted: hypertrophy, trabeculation, diverticuli Nodules may mimic carcinoma
Nodules within prostate: varied echogenicity (small—hypoechoic/large—hyperechoic) Color Doppler imaging demonstrates hypervascularity within or around nodules/masses Asymmetry of prostate Bulging margin of mass	Frequency of urination Urgency and feeling of constant fullness Hematuria Hematospermia Pain in pelvis, thighs, hips Labs: elevated PSA	Carcinoma of the prostate	Small tumors may not demonstrate flow with Doppler assessment Some tumors may be isoechoic and not detectable with sonography Guidance for prostate biopsy

Focal masses of varied echogenicity Calcifications and thickening of capsule may be noted	Fever Chills Pain Dysuria Hematuria Painful ejaculation	Chronic prostatitis	Associated with bacterial and nonbacterial causes

Solid mass projecting into the
  bladder lumen
	Painless hematuria	Bladder tumor
		  Papilloma
		  TCC
		  SCC
		  Metastatic
		Cystitis
		BPH
		Blood clots
		Endometriosis
			Most common cause is TCC
			Metastases from kidneys, uterus,
			  cervix, prostate, rectum

Patient Preparation

- Full bladder: 32 ounces of clear fluid before the examination; no voiding until after the examination is completed. Alternative: no preparation, TA imaging followed by endovaginal EV imaging.

Equipment and Technical Factors

- Curved linear, vector, linear array (for abdominal wall imaging), and EV transducers are used. The EV transducer should be adequately sheathed for the examination and appropriately disinfected after each use. Published guidelines for disinfection of endocavitary transducers are available. In addition, manufacturer specifications should be followed to avoid damaging the transducer.
- Color Doppler imaging can be used to distinguish vascular from nonvascular structures.

Imaging Protocol

- Longitudinal axis images through the medial, mid, and lateral aspects of the uterus and both adnexa. The endometrial thickness should be evaluated with the endometrium perpendicular to the beam (may be done by TA imaging, but EV imaging is more accurate).
- Transverse axis images through the cervix, body, and fundus of the uterus and both adnexa.
- Longitudinal and transverse axis images of the ovaries.
- EV imaging may be performed with the patient in the lithotomy position (gynecologic examination table with stirrups is preferred; a covered support wedge may be used to elevate hips) or the Sims position (useful when the patient is obese or cannot lie supine).
- Doppler evaluation of the ovaries will demonstrate variation in blood flow with menstrual cycle (resting versus ovulating ovary).
- Bimanual technique (external pressure over pelvic area) may place uterus and/or ovaries into the scan plane.

Measurements

Uterus (nulliparous)

- Length: 7.0 cm
- Width: 5.0 cm
- Thickness (AP): 3.0 cm

Uterus (multiparous)

- Approximately 2.0 cm larger in all three dimensions

Uterus (postpartum)

- Enlarged uterus should involute to multiparous size within 4 to 8 weeks after delivery

Uterus (postmenopausal)

- Length: 3.0–5.0 cm
- Width: 2.0–3.0 cm
- Depth (AP): 2.0–3.0 cm

Endometrial thickness

- Menstruating: 4.0–14.0 cm
- Postmenopausal: <5.0 mm

Ovary

- Length: 2.5–5.0 cm
- Postmenopausal: 5.8 cm^3
- Thickness (AP): 0.6–2.2 cm
- Width: 1.5–3.0 cm

Ovarian volume 0.523 (L × W × D)

Menstruating: 9.8 cm^3

Female Pelvis

Sonographic Finding(s)	Clinical Presentation	Differential Diagnosis	Next Step
Anechoic structure(s) in cervix	Asymptomatic	Nabothian cyst(s)	Document size and location
Enlarged, bulky uterus with distinct mass(es) noted	Uterus enlarged on manual examination	Leiomyoma (fibroid/myoma)	Intramural fibroids may displace endometrial canal without change in overall uterine shape
Possibly heterogenous echotexture without identification of specific mass(es)	Asymptomatic to mild symptoms	Intramural Subserosal Pedunculated	Subserosal fibroids distort contour of uterus even when small
Possible irregular border	Common complaints: feeling of pelvic "fullness" or pressure, back pain, urinary incontinence, painful periods	All types may demonstrate necrosis and degeneration	Pedunculated fibroids may not demonstrate connecting stalk
Hypoechoic, hyperechoic, heterogenous, or complex mass(es); small to very large in size		All types may enlarge during pregnancy and regress after menopause	Evaluate urinary bladder for impingement by uterus
Possible calcification within mass(es)		Adenomyosis	

Possible displacement of
  endometrial canal
Hydronephrosis/hydroureter
  may be noted

Normal size uterus with focal thickening or distortion of endometrium	Heavy bleeding during periods, may interfere with fertility Labs: decreased hematocrit; anemia (if bleeding is heavy and prolonged)	Leiomyoma Submucosal Endometrial polyp Intramural fibroid	Sonohysterogram to reveal true endometrial thickness and confirm presence of submucosal fibroid or polyp 3D imaging may be helpful Fibroid may prolapse into vagina
Ovarian cyst, <2.5 cm in diameter	Asymptomatic	Dominant follicle (menstruating women) Postmenopausal woman: suspicious for ovarian carcinoma	Serial sonograms should demonstrate change in cyst with menstruation

continued

Female Pelvis—*cont'd*

Sonographic Finding(s)	Clinical Presentation	Differential Diagnosis	Next Step
Ovarian cyst, 3.0 cm to 20.0 cm Possible internal echoes	Asymptomatic Pelvic pain if cyst is large Hemorrhage may cause fever, pain Dysfunctional uterine bleeding if cyst produces hormones	Follicular cyst	Internal echoes may indicate hemorrhage Large cyst may cause ovarian torsion
Uterine body and fundus are the same size as cervix	Asymptomatic	Menopausal woman: normal atrophy of uterus Prepubertal uterus	Size and appearance of ovaries should correlate with uterus
Enlarged uterus with bulbous fundus Uterus is hypoechoic and heterogenous	Painful vaginal bleeding Heavy bleeding	Adenomyosis Diffuse/focal Leiomyoma	Most commonly found in multiparous women

Anterior or posterior wall may be eccentrically enlarged Small cysts in myometrium Multiple areas of attenuation		Myometrial contraction Endometrial carcinoma	
Rapid enlargement of fibroid Hydroureter hydronephrosis may be noted	Possible rapid increase in abdominal girth	Leiomyosarcoma	Evaluate urinary bladder for impingement by uterus
Bulky, enlarged cervix	Asymptomatic Labs: positive PAP smear	Cervical carcinoma Cervical myoma	Evaluate urinary bladder for impingement by cervix
Two uterine horns, two cervices, two vaginas	Asymptomatic Uterus enlarged on manual examination Heavy periods	Uterus didelphys	Associated with renal anomalies and pregnancy complications

continued

Female Pelvis—*cont'd*

Sonographic Finding(s)	Clinical Presentation	Differential Diagnosis	Next Step
Two uterine horns noted (two endometria)	Asymptomatic Uterus enlarged on manual examination Heavy periods	Uterus bicornis	Associated with renal anomalies and pregnancy complications
Two endometrial stripes are noted Appearance of divided endometrium	Asymptomatic Possible uterine enlargement on manual examination	Uterus subseptus	Associated with renal anomalies and pregnancy complications
Narrow uterine fundus	Asymptomatic Uterus smaller than normal on manual examination	Uterus unicornis	Associated with renal anomalies and pregnancy complications

Endometrial thickness >14.0 mm; may be diffuse or focal Menstrual age or postmenopausal woman on HRT	Unexplained vaginal bleeding Heavy or long periods Labs: decreased hematocrit	Normal secretory endometrium Early pregnancy Endometrial hyperplasia Endometrial carcinoma	Consistent thickness: endometrial hyperplasia or polyp(s) Postmenopausal woman: suspect endometrial carcinoma Evaluate endometrial blood flow
Endometrial thickness >4.0 mm; may be diffuse or focal	Vaginal bleeding Postmenopausal Labs: decreased hematocrit if bleeding is heavy	Endometrial hyperplasia Endometrial carcinoma	Risk of endometrial carcinoma increases with thickness of 20.0 mm, fluid, and uterine enlargement Increased endometrial blood flow is associated with carcinoma *continued*

Female Pelvis—cont'd

Sonographic Finding(s)	Clinical Presentation	Differential Diagnosis	Next Step
Fluid collection in endometrium	Asymptomatic Unexplained vaginal bleeding History of infertility Labs: decreased hematocrit if collection is related to bleeding	Small collection: menstruation, ectopic pregnancy, endometritis, degenerating fibroid, decidual reaction, recent abortion, Asherman's syndrome Large collection: cervical stenosis, cancer in any part of reproductive tract, endometrial hyperplasia or polyp(s), congenital anomalies	Life-threatening condition if ectopic pregnancy is suspected or patient has undergone a recent abortion
Dilated hypoechoic thick-walled fallopian tube(s) with tapering at uterine cornu	Pelvic pain Fever Nausea	Pyosalpinx (tube filled with pus; active infection)	Evaluate for presence of abscess

Indistinct posterior border of uterus Possible fluid in posterior cul-de-sac and Morison's pouch	Vomiting Chills Dyspareunia Cervical pain or tenderness on manual examination Labs: elevated WBC; positive vaginal cultures for *Chlamydia* or gonorrhea	Bilateral: feature of PID Unilateral: feature of extended infection from bowel or surgery	
Dilated anechoic thin-walled fallopian tube(s) Tapering at uterine cornu Determined NOT to be dilated veins on color Doppler imaging	Asymptomatic Some colicky pelvic pain or lower abdominal tenderness History of bowel infection or surgery Labs: positive vaginal cultures for *Chlamydia* or gonorrhea	Hydrosalpinx (closed off fallopian tube) Bilateral: feature of PID (resolved pyosalpinx) Unilateral: extended infection from bowel or surgery *or* strictures from pelvic previous surgery	Immobile pelvic structures (ovaries are fixed in position) indicate presence of adhesions from infection or surgery

continued

Female Pelvis—*cont'd*

Sonographic Finding(s)	Clinical Presentation	Differential Diagnosis	Next Step
Unilateral or bilateral thick-walled complex "masses" in pelvis; possible fluid levels Blurring of pelvic tissue planes (indistinct organs) Possible fluid in posterior cul-de-sac and Morison's pouch EV imaging may not be tolerable	Severe lower abdominal and pelvic pain Severe cervical pain on manipulation Nausea Vomiting RUQ pain Labs: elevated WBC; positive vaginal cultures for *Chlamydia* or gonorrhea	Tubo-ovarian abscess Bilateral: feature/sequel of PID Unilateral: possible extension of other infection	Peritonitis is a life-threatening complication May require invasive procedure to resolve
Ovarian cyst, <4.0 cm with thick walls and internal echoes Increased flow noted with color Doppler imaging	Asymptomatic Pelvic pain (hemorrhage) Labs: increased progesterone	Corpus luteum cyst	In pregnancy corpus luteum should not persist after 16 weeks' gestation May need serial scans to follow regression

Large swollen ovary (>4.0 cm) Hypoechoic to hyperechoic Tiny follicles around "mass" Free fluid in cul-de-sac Doppler imaging may show decreased or absent flow (nonspecific finding)	Severe lower abdominal pain Nausea Vomiting Fever More common in RLQ and in young girls and women	Ovarian torsion Complete Partial	Related to ovarian enlargement, cyst, tumor May mimic pain from ectopic pregnancy
Cyst adjacent to but separate from ovary No change in size of this cyst with serial sonograms May hemorrhage or undergo torsion	Adnexal mass felt during manual examination No complaints unless hemorrhage or torsion occur	Paraovarian cyst (located in broad ligament) Peritoneal inclusion cyst (remnant of surgery)	Demonstrate that cyst is separate ovary

continued

Female Pelvis—*cont'd*

Sonographic Finding(s)	Clinical Presentation	Differential Diagnosis	Next Step
Unilateral "mass" in adnexa/ pelvis found in woman of childbearing age May be solid, predominately solid or predominately cystic With/without calcifications Strong near field echogenicity with loss of sound penetration (tip-of-the-iceberg appearance)	Asymptomatic Pelvic fullness or lower abdominal pressure Possible incidental finding during radiographic procedure Labs: elevated AFP in approximately 50% of patients (immature teratoma)	Cystic dermoid/mature teratoma Presence of germ cell tissue: hair, bone, fat (predominately ectoderm) Immature teratoma is more rapid growing	Unable to differentiate benign from malignant (immature teratoma) with sonography Low occurrence of bilateral findings Color Doppler imaging may demonstrate flow in wall of mass
Thick walled "cyst" in adnexa (possible bilateral) in woman of menstruating age; may appear "solid" but no acoustic shadowing	Asymptomatic *or* Intense chronic pelvic pain Infertility	Endometrioma (chocolate cyst) Hemorrhagic ovarian cyst	Presence and size of endometrioma is unrelated to severity of endometriosis Rupture results in acute abdomen

Possible ovarian enlargement May mimic hemorrhagic ovarian cyst or abscess		Dermoid Ovarian neoplasm	
Normal to enlarged ovaries with small follicles around periphery	Asymptomatic Anovulation Amenorrhea Infertility Hirsutism Obesity Labs: elevated LH; low FSH level; abnormal estrogen and progesterone	PCOS Multiple ovarian follicular cysts Polycystic ovaries (normal hormone levels)	Associated with Stein- Leventhal syndrome (PCOS)
Bilateral large multiple cysts; ovarian tissue difficult to discern because of multiple large cysts Ascites and pleural effusion may be noted	Pain Elevated blood pressure Labs: extremely high β-hCG level	Theca lutein cysts	Associated with OHS (also called OHSS) or molar pregnancy

continued

Female Pelvis—*cont'd*

Sonographic Finding(s)	Clinical Presentation	Differential Diagnosis	Next Step
Large cystic/complex structure in adnexa; irregular thin/thick walls with/without papillary projections Possible septations/loculations Large: mass may extend into abdomen; prone to torsion Possible bilateral, usually unilateral Color Doppler imaging demonstrates flow in solid portions of structure	Asymptomatic Increasing abdominal girth Pelvic pain (torsion) Leg edema from IVC compression Labs: elevated CA 125, estrogen or progesterone	Benign: cystadenoma (serous more common than mucinous) Malignant: cystadenocarcinoma (serous more common than mucinous) Endometrioid (malignant, associated with endometriosis)	IVC compression and metastatic disease may be present Mucinous may produce hormones; more common to have thick walls; may cause more symptoms; may rupture, causing pseudomyxoma peritonei Serous has more papillary projections

Small, hypoechoic mass noted on ovary Calcifications may be present May be bilateral	Asymptomatic *or* May have abnormal vaginal bleeding or increasing abdominal size Labs: abnormal estrogen level	Brenner tumor (transitional cell tumor)	Commonly an incidental finding Associated with Meigs' syndrome
Large, solid mass on ovary Prone to torsion More common in older (menopausal) women	Asymptomatic Torsion Meigs' syndrome Abnormal vaginal bleeding	Fibroma (nonfunctioning) Thecoma (produces estrogen)	Locate and document ascites Evaluate thorax for pleural effusion
Large (5.0–15.0 cm) unilateral complex (multiloculated/cystic) mass found in younger woman (most commonly found in 20- to 30-year-olds)	Amenorrhea Infertility Pelvic discomfort if very large Labs: increased testosterone level	Sertoli-Leydig cell tumor (arrhenoblastoma or androblastoma)	Masculinizing tumor

continued

Female Pelvis—*cont'd*

Sonographic Finding(s)	Clinical Presentation	Differential Diagnosis	Next Step
Unilateral, cystic, or solid mass on ovary Menstruating or menopausal woman May be large (12.0 cm) May undergo torsion or rupture (severe pain)	Pelvic pain Dysfunctional uterine bleeding Uterine enlargement Breast enlargement and tenderness Labs: increased estrogen	Granulosa cell tumor Endometrioma Cystadenoma	Feminizing tumor Low-grade malignancy Some association with endometrial carcinoma
Unilateral solid mass in young woman Calcifications, areas of necrosis may be seen	Elevated BP Nausea Vomiting Labs: elevated β-hCG; elevated AFP	Dysgerminoma Teratoma Epithelial ovarian tumor	Germ cell tumor more common in early reproductive years Enlarged lymph nodes may be present
Complex or solid mass in adnexa (may be bilateral) in menopausal woman	Abdominal pain and swelling Indigestion Frequent urination Constipation	Primary ovarian malignancy	50% are advanced when found

May be large or small; may extend beyond ovary Ovarian enlargement may be noted Ascites	Weight gain from ascites Family history of breast or ovarian cancer Labs: elevated CA 125 (nonspecific)	Most common are epithelial tumors: serous/mucinous cystadenocarcinoma, endometrioid Less common are germ cell tumors, stromal tumors	Evaluate for enlarged lymph nodes, spread to ipsilateral ovary, liver Doppler evaluation of ovary may demonstrate increased flow
Bilateral solid/complex ovarian masses May mimic any type of ovarian mass Ascites	History of primary carcinoma: bowel, breast, endometrium, melanoma, lymphoma Abdominal swelling (ascites) Weight loss Abnormal labs related to primary disease	Metastatic ovarian tumor	Bilateral tumors strongly associated with metastatic disease Kruckenberg's tumor: metastases from bowel

OBSTETRICS

Patient Preparation

- Preparation is similar to that for the female pelvis; however, an extremely full bladder may compress the gestational sac. Alternative: no preparation. TA imaging followed by EV imaging may be done.

Equipment and Technical Factors

- MI and TI settings must comply with the ALARA principle; pulsed-wave Doppler imaging should not be used during the first trimester to obtain an EHR because of the high intensity than can be focused on the developing heart.
- If there is difficulty locating the embryonic heart with 2D imaging, color or power Doppler imaging may be used sparingly to locate the heart for M-mode cursor placement.
- Doppler imaging may be used in the evaluation of adnexal pathologic conditions.

Imaging Protocol

- Longitudinal axis images through the medial, mid, and lateral aspects of the uterus should include the gestational sac; include images of both adnexa and ovaries.
- The gestational sac should be evaluated for the presence of absence of an embryo, early placenta, and membranes (EV imaging provides the best resolution).
- Transverse axis images through the cervix, body, and fundus of the uterus should include the gestational sac; include images of both adnexa and ovaries.
- Appropriate measurements are performed: MSD and CRL of the embryo; the yolk sac diameter may be obtained.
- Compare measurements obtained during the sonographic examination with the date of the patient's last menstrual period and the estimated delivery date.

- The EHR should be documented with use of M-mode imaging.
- Near the end of the first trimester, fetal biometry may be obtained.

Measurements

Gestational Sac

- Calculate the MSD $(L + W + D)/3$; correlate with patient's dates; accuracy is +1 week.

CRL

- Accuracy +3 days; refer to published charts (see Appendix A).

Yolk sac

- Maximum diameter: 5.0–6.0 cm

Nuchal translucency at 9–13 weeks (45.0 mm–84.0 mm CRL)

- <3.0 mm

- MSD and CRL measurements can be referenced to standard charts and recorded on a technical worksheet if software package is not available.
- The location and size of a uterine fibroid should be documented during each sonogram of the pregnancy.

First Trimester

Sonographic Finding(s)	Clinical Presentation	Differential Diagnosis	Next Step
No yolk sac noted in a gestational sac <10.0 mm (EV scanning) No embryo noted in a gestational sac <18.0 mm (EV scanning) Irregular sac with lack of decidual reaction Sac is low in uterus	Pregnancy "feels different"; diminished morning sickness and breast tenderness Vaginal bleeding Cramping Advanced maternal age Diabetes History of recurrent abortions Labs: positive β-hCG	Anembryonic pregnancy (blighted ovum) Normal intrauterine pregnancy Pseudosac (ectopic pregnancy)	Serial β-hCG and sonograms may be done May require surgical intervention to resolve
Yolk sac measures <6.0 cm with/without presence of embryo	Asymptomatic	Enlarged yolk sac	Associated with pregnancy loss

Ovarian cyst, <4.0 cm with thick walls and internal echoes Increased flow noted with color Doppler imaging	Asymptomatic Hemorrhage may cause pain Labs: increased progesterone	Corpus luteum cyst	Should not persist after 16 weeks' gestation May need serial scans to follow regression
Cystic area in posterior fetal brain noted at 8–11 weeks' gestation	Asymptomatic	Normal rhombencephalon (hindbrain)	Precursor to fourth ventricle
Protrusion or bulge at umbilical cord insertion into embryo/fetus noted at 8–12 weeks' gestation	Asymptomatic	Normal physiological gut/umbilical herniation Early omphalocele	Should regress by 12 weeks' gestation Early omphalocele persists after 12 weeks' gestation *continued*

First Trimester—*cont'd*

Sonographic Finding(s)	Clinical Presentation	Differential Diagnosis	Next Step
Nuchal translucency measurement >3.0 mm seen between 9 and 13.8 weeks' gestation (45.0 mm–84.0 mm CRL)	Asymptomatic Screening exam Labs: abnormal PAPP-A	Increased nuchal translucency	Accuracy of measurement is critical Associated with numerous genetic and nongenetic abnormalities/defects and cardiac defects
Anechoic space between amnion and chorion at 12 weeks' gestation	Asymptomatic	Normal chorioamniotic separation	Chorion and amnion may not fuse until 16 weeks' gestation
Single gestation with adjacent empty gestational sac or anechoic area/structure	Asymptomatic Vaginal spotting or bleeding	Subchorionic/ perigestational hemorrhage Loss of dichorionic twin ("vanishing" twin)	Hemorrhage will follow the shape of the viable gestational sac

Crescent-shaped fluid collection noted between gestational sac and uterine wall	Vaginal spotting or bleeding Cramping Closed cervix	Threatened abortion Subchorionic/ perigestational hemorrhage Marginal placental hematoma (asymptomatic)	Pregnancy may have normal outcome *or* Large/extensive hematoma may lead to spontaneous abortion
Gestational sac is low in uterus and may be bulging into cervix or upper vagina Cervical funneling may be seen Gestational sac may be small	Bleeding Passing clots Cramping Leakage of fluid Labs: plateau of β-hCG level	Abortion in progress Also known as: inevitable/impending abortion	Associated with cervical incompetence and pregnancy loss
Collapsed and misshapened gestational sac	Bleeding Passing clots or tissue Cramping Leakage of fluid	Incomplete abortion (progression of a threatened or inevitable abortion) *continued*	Retention of some products of conception

First Trimester—*cont'd*

Sonographic Finding(s)	Clinical Presentation	Differential Diagnosis	Next Step
Thickened endometrium with/without evidence of retained fetal parts	Labs: slow fall or plateau of β-hCG level		
Intact gestational sac with nonviable embryo/fetus Evidence of hydropic change of placenta may be noted	Asymptomatic *or* Uterus small for dates	Missed abortion Embryonic/fetal death	Unexpected finding; use care and tact in dealing with patient
No evidence of gestational sac; "empty" uterus Thickened endometrial line may be present	Uterus is enlarged Bleeding Cramping Labs: rapid fall of β-hCG	Complete abortion Early intrauterine pregnancy (β-hCG levels should rise)	Echoes in uterus may represent blood rather than retained products of conception Serial sonograms may be needed to confirm diagnosis

EHR/FHR less than normal for stage of gestation Heart rate of <90 beats/min	Asymptomatic	Bradycardia	Associated with pregnancy loss
Two complete gestational sacs, each with a yolk sac or embryo/fetus Gestational sacs are separated by thick membrane or tissue	Asymptomatic *or* Hyperemesis Uterus measures large for dates	Dichorionic/diamniotic gestation	Embryos may be same or opposite sex: early division of fertilized ovum (MZ) or fertilization of two separate ova (DZ) Associated with complications of pregnancy (hypertension, placenta previa or abruptio placentae, hemorrhage), preterm delivery, IUGR, and fetal anomalies compared with singleton pregnancy *continued*

First Trimester—*cont'd*

Sonographic Finding(s)	Clinical Presentation	Differential Diagnosis	Next Step
Single gestational sac containing two amniotic sacs, each with a yolk sac or embryo/fetus Membranes are thin	Asymptomatic *or* Hyperemesis Uterus measures large for dates	Monochorionic/diamniotic gestation (MZ:MC/DA)	Embryos always the same sex Single placenta Associated with development of TTTS, TRAP, TES; pregnancy loss
Single gestational sac with no separating membrane between yolk sacs or embryos/fetuses	Asymptomatic *or* Hyperemesis Uterus measures large for dates	Monochorionic/monoamniotic gestation (MZ:MC/MA)	Embryos always the same sex Single placenta Associated with fetal anomalies and development of locking twins, TTTS, polyhydramnios; pregnancy loss

Single gestational sac with no separating membrane between yolk sacs or embryos/fetuses Embryos/fetuses cannot be separated or appear to join at the chest, abdomen, or head Fused or multiple vessels in umbilical cord	Asymptomatic *or* Hyperemesis Uterus measures large for dates	Conjoined twins (MZ:MC/MA)	Division of zygote >13 days post conception Associated with multiple fetal anomalies (sharing of structures), fetal death or stillborn
No evidence of intrauterine gestational sac with discriminatory β-hCG level of 800–1000 mIU/ml (2nd IS) or 1000–2000 mIU/ml (IRP) Fluid collection in endometrium (pseudogestational sac)	Pain or discomfort Bleeding, possibly heavy Possible pelvic mass on manual exam History of ectopic pregnancy, prior tubal surgery, PID, or infertility	Ectopic pregnancy Normal early IUP with/without corpus luteum cyst	Correct gain settings to detect echoes within fluid (evidence of blood) Adnexal mass or echogenic ring may be mistaken for corpus luteum cyst Pseudosac can mimic normal IUP *continued*

First Trimester—cont'd

Sonographic Finding(s)	Clinical Presentation	Differential Diagnosis	Next Step
Eccentric fundal location of gestational sac: endometrial line seen as separate structure <5.0 mm of myometrium surrounding sac	Pelvic or abdominal pain Hypotension Shock Labs: normal doubling of β-hCG	Interstitial/cornual ectopic pregnancy Adnexal ectopic pregnancy	Life-threatening finding: high risk of rupture and hemorrhage
Decidual reaction (thick endometrium) Mass in adnexa (adnexal ring) may or may not be noted Fluid (with/without echoes) may be noted in posterior cul-de-sac or Morison's pouch (rupture) May be bilateral	Labs: β-hCG level may plateau or be subnormal		Color Doppler imaging can demonstrate "ring of fire" appearance even if gray scale fails to demonstrate adnexal mass (can mimic corpus luteum cyst)

| Live intrauterine pregnancy and adnexal ectopic mass | Pain or discomfort
Bleeding, possibly heavy
History of prior tubal surgery, PID, or infertility
Labs: βhCG level may be normal or elevated | Heterotopic pregnancy | Rare
Associated with ovulation induction and in vitro fertilization |

Patient Preparation

- No voiding immediately before the examination; some fluid in the bladder is needed to visualize the urinary bladder and may aid in visualization of the cervix and LUS.

Equipment and Technical Factors

- A curved linear transducer is commonly used. An EV transducer may be used to visualize the cervix and LUS, or the presence of a pathologic condition must be more clearly documented; ensure that the department protocols are followed. EV imaging may be contraindicated in the presence of vaginal bleeding, leakage of fluid, or cervical dilation.
- Fetal, uterine, or ovarian Doppler imaging may be performed as requested; Doppler imaging may be used in the evaluation of pathologic conditions found during the study.
- MI and TI settings must comply with the ALARA principle.

Imaging Protocol

- Determine the location of the placenta and the fetal lie; assess the presence of pathologic conditions or anatomical variants.
  The presence and location of fibroid(s) should be documented.
  The ovaries and adnexal areas should be evaluated.
- Braxton-Hicks contractions may occur throughout pregnancy. This type of contraction usually lasts 20 to 30 minutes and can occur in any area of the uterus (may mimic fibroid, placenta previa, or mass).

Minimum documentation images

- Placenta: sagittal plane images through the medial, mid, and lateral aspects of the uterus; transverse plane images through the cervix, body, and fundus.
- Length and diameter of the cervix (perform immediately after patient lies on scan table; use TA, transperineal, or EV imaging to clearly demonstrate cervix (follow department protocols in using EV imaging).

- Umbilical cord insertion into placenta and fetus; three-vessel cord in transverse axis. The amount of amniotic fluid should be documented and assessed.

Fetal anatomy to include:

Posterior fossa for cisterna magna and nuchal thickness

Lateral ventricles and cerebral hemispheres

Profile for forehead shape, nose, mouth, and chin

Nose and mouth using a coronal plane

Spine: cervical, thoracic, and lumbar

Thorax to include the heart: apical long axis, parasternal long axis, short axis and outflow tracts: heart rate documented with M mode

Abdomen to include the stomach, liver, intrahepatic portal vein, kidneys, urinary bladder, bowel, and fetal umbilical cord insertion

Extremities; confirm two complete upper and lower

Sex (check department protocols)

- Biophysical profile 30 minutes; scoring: 2 = meets all criteria or 0 = did not meet criteria:

Fetal breathing: one episode lasting 30 seconds

Gross body movements: three trunk or limb movements

Fetal tone: one extension and flexion of limb or trunk

Amniotic fluid volume: single pocket of 2.0 cm in AP dimension

Measurements

- The uterus is generally not measured during pregnancy; however, fibroid size should be documented.

Fetal biometry (BPD, HC, AC, FL)

- Compare measurements obtained (recommend average of three of each required measurement) with patient's estimated due date and standardized charts or use the equipment software.

Other

- Thorax/abdomen: 1:1 ratio
- Occipital-frontal diameter/BPD $\times$ 100: CI to correlate with BPD

- Ventricular atrium: <1 cm
- Cisterna magna: 5.0–10.0 mm
- Nuchal translucency at 9–13 weeks: <3.0 mm
- Nuchal thickness at 16–22 weeks: <6.0 mm
- Amniotic fluid: Amniotic fluid index (AP dimension of four quadrants = 5.0–24.0 cm)
- Single pocket (AP dimension = 2.0–8.0 cm)
- Ocular diameter
- All long bones

Second and Third Trimester Fetus

Sonographic Finding(s)	Clinical Presentation	Differential Diagnosis	Next Step
Two or more of the following are noted: Ascites Pleural effusion Pericardial effusion Edema Placentomegaly Polyhydramnios	Uterus is large for dates Rh sensitized (immune hydrops/fetal anemia)	Hydrops fetalis Isolated ascites, pleural effusion, pericardial effusion	Nonimmune causes include maternal infection, chromosomal abnormalities (especially Turner's syndrome, trisomies 13, 18, and 21), and heart failure Associated with fetal tachycardia Elevated PSV from the MCA associated with immune hydrops *continued*

Second and Third Trimester Fetus—*cont'd*

Sonographic Finding(s)	Clinical Presentation	Differential Diagnosis	Next Step
Fetal biometry: all measurements (including weight) are below 10th percentile for gestational age Fetal soft tissues may appear thin Placenta may appear thin and small Oligohydramnios (especially in late pregnancy) may be present	Uterus measures small for dates Previous sonogram demonstrated below normal or normal fetal gestational age	Symmetric IUGR Wrong dates SGA fetus	Associated with both chromosomal and nonchromosomal abnormalities BPP score, umbilical artery Doppler, or S/D ratio may be abnormal if this is true symmetric IUGR Symmetric IUGR requires at least two sets of biometry to confirm finding
Fetal abdomen measures below 10th percentile for gestational age but head and femur measurements are within normal limits for gestational age	Uterus measures appropriately or small for dates Previous sonogram demonstrated normal fetal measurements for gestational age	Asymmetric IUGR	Placental insufficiency may be documented by Doppler interrogation of umbilical artery MCA S/D ratio < umbilical artery S/D ratio Pulsatile flow in umbilical vein

Placenta may demonstrate aging (grade 3 or 4) early in pregnancy Oligohydramnios Echogenic bowel may be noted	Maternal diabetes or hypertension before pregnancy		
Fetal biometry reveals fetal abdominal measurement above 90th percentile for gestational age Evidence of skin thickening around fetal head and trunk; prominent fetal cheeks	Uterus measures large for dates Commonly seen in cases of maternal diabetes, obesity, advanced maternal age, and multiparity	Macrosomia	In suspected macrosomia, carefully scan the anatomy to document size of fetal liver and to search for anomalies such as GI tract, cardiovascular system (thickening of the cardiac IVS), CNS, and VACTERL
Possible mild polyhydramnios may be present			Increased size of facial cheeks is due to fat deposits Placenta usually demonstrates increased thickness

Second and Third Trimester Fetal Head and Neck

Sonographic Finding(s)	Clinical Presentation	Differential Diagnosis	Next Step
Unable to obtain BPD/no skull is visible Fetal face has "mask" or "frog-face" appearance Polyhydramnios	Uterus may measure large for dates	Anencephaly	Associated with CNS and other anomalies, hydronephrosis, diaphragmatic hernia, cleft lip, and cardiac anomalies; may also be caused by amniotic band
Cerebellar hemispheres lack rounded appearance; unable to visualize cerebellum Asymmetrical ventriculomegaly (third and lateral ventricles) with splaying of lateral ventricles; small cranial size Skull demonstrates depression of frontal bones	Asymptomatic	Chiari type II	Associated with spina bifida and agenesis of the corpus callosum Normal frontal bones may demonstrate slight depression

Third ventricle is seen more superior in midline of brain Lateral ventricles are seen more lateral and parallel to midline Mild ventriculomegaly A communicating cyst may be seen superior to the third ventricle Gyri are more vertically aligned and appear to radiate from lateral ventricles Possible polyhydramnios	Asymptomatic	Agenesis of corpus callosum	Associated with several anomalies: Dandy-Walker syndrome, holoprosence-phaly, medial facial clefts, encephalocele, or meningo-myelocele, trisomy 8, 13, and 18, diaphragmatic hernia, cardiac malformations, missing or small lung(s), and renal agenesis or dysplasia
Lateral ventricle(s) appear prominent BPD and HC within normal limits for gestational age Ventricular atrium measures >10.0 mm in AP diameter Choroid plexus may appear to "dangle" within dilated ventricular atrium	Asymptomatic	Ventriculomegaly	Associated with aqueductal stenosis Normal choroids should fill ventricular atrium or there should be no more than a 3-mm gap between choroid plexus and ventricle wall *continued*

Second and Third Trimester Fetal Head and Neck—*cont'd*

Sonographic Finding(s)	Clinical Presentation	Differential Diagnosis	Next Step
Ventricles (lateral and third, possibly fourth) and fetal head size are enlarged Brain mantle may appear thin Falx is intact Abnormal orbits, face, feet, and hands Polyhydramnios	Uterus may measure large for dates	Hydrocephalus	Indicates presence of obstruction (noncommunicating) in ventricular system or may be related to aqueductal stenosis, meningomyelocele, spina bifida, encephalocele, or Dandy-Walker malformation, trisomy 13 or 18 Document level or point of obstruction if possible
Ventriculomegaly (lateral and third; fourth ventricle is normal) with intact falx and preservation of brain mantle Cerebellum and cisterna magna appear normal	Exposure to teratogens or cytomegalovirus Maternal history of toxoplasmosis or syphilis	Aqueductal stenosis	Causes 35.7% of hydrocephalus and is more common in males (X linked) In utero infections or intracranial tumor may be underlying cause

			Mild ventriculomegaly has been associated with trisomy 21
Large cyst in posterior fossa with normal fourth ventricle not seen Posterior fossa is enlarged Vermis of cerebellum is not seen and hemispheres may appear splayed and flattened Possible ventriculomegaly or hydrocephalus and agenesis of corpus callosum Possible polyhydramnios	Uterus may measure large for dates	Dandy-Walker malformation Enlarged cisterna magna	Associated with both intracranial and extracranial abnormalities: agenesis of corpus callosum, facial clefts, CNS, and cardiac ventricular septal defect, trisomy 13, 18, or 21 May be seen in Meckel-Gruber syndrome
Irregular cystic structure(s) noted adjacent to lateral ventricle(s); may show connection to lateral ventricle	Maternal thrombocytopenia, anticoagulation therapy, drug use such as cocaine; trauma	Porencephalic cyst	Rare: This finding is a result of resolved hemorrhage in parenchyma Associated with TTTS and death of a cotwin

continued

Second and Third Trimester Fetal Head and Neck—*cont'd*

Sonographic Finding(s)	Clinical Presentation	Differential Diagnosis	Next Step
Fetal skull is enlarged and demonstrates bulge from top of head Polyhydramnios	Uterus may measure large for dates	Cloverleaf skull	Associated with thanatophoric dysplasia, Apert syndrome, or amniotic band
Sac/mass protrudes from occipital portion of fetal skull If the sac/mass is large, microcephaly may be present Hydrocephalus may be seen Microcephaly or depressed frontal bones of the skull may be noted	Asymptomatic Labs: MSAFP may be elevated	Encephalocele	Associated with Meckel-Gruber syndrome, polydactyly, polycystic kidneys, liver cysts, cleft palate, and cardiac anomalies An encephalocele found on the lateral aspect of the head may be caused by amniotic band Large encephaloceles can cause microcephaly or depressed frontal cranial bones

Unable to identify normal fetal orbits	Maternal history of toxoplasmosis or rubella	Microphthalmia Anophthalmia	May be a sporadic anomaly, a result of in utero infection, trisomy 18, or Meckel-Gruber syndrome
Eyes are widely spaced	Asymptomatic	Hypertelorism	May represent familial trait or may be related to presence of frontal encephalocele, Noonan or Crouzon syndrome
Eyes are closely spaced	Asymptomatic	Hypotelorism	May represent familial trait or may be related to presence of holoprosencephaly, trisomy 13 or 18, or Meckel-Gruber syndrome *continued*

Second and Third Trimester Fetal Head and Neck—*cont'd*

Sonographic Finding(s)	Clinical Presentation	Differential Diagnosis	Next Step
Single orbit is seen	Asymptomatic	Cyclopia	Strongly associated with holoprosencephaly
Fetal chin is absent or difficult to see Possible polyhydramnios	Uterus may measure large for dates	Micrognathia	Associated with trisomy 18 and less commonly with trisomy 13 Also may be seen in other syndromes and skeletal dysplasias/ dystoses
Large midline fluid-filled space with thin rim of brain tissue Falx may or may not be present Thalamus appears fused May demonstrate univentricle (horseshoe-shaped ventricle); hydrocephalus	Uterus may measure large for dates	Holoprosencephaly Alobar Semilobar Lobar	Difficult to differentiate semilobar from alobar Associated findings: clubfoot, omphalocele, IUGR, and features of trisomy 13, 18, Meckel-Gruber syndrome

Agenesis of the corpus callosum, cleft lip/palate may be noted Hypotelorism or cyclopia and proboscis may be seen			May mimic hydranencephaly
Large, fluid-filled cranium with cerebellum and midbrain seen No brain mantle seen Polyhydramnios	Uterus may measure large for dates	Hydranencephaly Massive hydrocephalus	Falx may or may not be intact May mimic alobar holoprosencephaly
A gap in soft tissue between the upper lip and nose (unilateral and bilateral) Sweeping coronal scan plane posteriorly through fetal mouth may reveal gap in bones of upper palate Polyhydramnios May be unilateral or bilateral	Uterus may measure large for dates	Cleft lip with/without cleft palate	Isolated or may be associated with midline cranial defects such as holoprosencephaly (midline clefts) or anencephaly Cleft lip and palate are seen in fetuses with chromosomal defects More commonly seen in male fetuses *continued*

Second and Third Trimester Fetal Head and Neck—*cont'd*

Sonographic Finding(s)	Clinical Presentation	Differential Diagnosis	Next Step
Fetal tongue protrudes from mouth at all times Polyhydramnios	Uterus may measure large for dates Maternal diabetes	Macroglossia	Associated with Beckwith-Wiedemann syndrome, trisomy 21, omphalocele, organomegaly Oral mass that is displacing tongue may be present
A cyst or cystic structures seen on the posterior aspect or surrounding fetal neck Placenta may be large and edematous Hydrops	Uterus may measure large for dates Labs: MSAFP may be lower or higher than normal	Cystic hygroma Teratoma Neural tube defect Hemangioma	Associated with Turner syndrome (45,X) and trisomy 13, 18, or 21 Note: Cystic hygromas are most commonly found in the neck but can occur in the axilla, groin, or mediastinum

Second and Third Trimester Fetal Thorax and Heart

Sonographic Finding(s)	Clinical Presentation	Differential Diagnosis	Next Step
Fetal thorax appears narrow Thorax to abdomen ratio is below 1:1 Polyhydramnios (skeletal disorders) *or* Oligohydramnios (renal agenesis)	Uterus measures small or large for dates	Lethal dwarfism Pulmonary hypoplasia	Associated with many skeletal dysplasias and dystoses: thanatophoric dysplasia, achondrogenesis, and osteogenesis imperfecta type II Also related to lack of lung development related to renal agenesis
Cystic structure in thorax, possibly displacing the heart Polyhydramnios	Uterus may measure large for dates	Bronchogenic cyst	Document stomach inferior to diaphragm; if stomach is not seen in the normal location, the "cyst" may be the stomach: diaphragmatic hernia *continued*

Second and Third Trimester Fetal Thorax and Heart—*cont'd*

Sonographic Finding(s)	Clinical Presentation	Differential Diagnosis	Next Step
Fluid is seen to surround one or both lungs Fluid around left lung may displace heart to right side Thorax may measure larger than normal Polyhydramnios	Uterus may measure large for dates	Pleural effusion	Isolated finding or associated with fetal hydrops Massive effusions may lead to pulmonary hypoplasia
Significant fluid is seen around heart Polyhydramnios	Uterus may measure large for dates	Pericardial effusion	Isolated finding or may be associated with fetal hydrops, cardiac anomaly, arrhythmia, fetal anemia May compress heart Some fluid around heart may be normal

Right side of heart appears more prominent with wall thickening Unable to obtain symmetrical four-chamber view of heart	Asymptomatic	Hypoplastic left heart	Isolated finding or part of a complex or syndrome
Cardiac septum appears to have "gaps" between atria or ventricles	Asymptomatic	ASD/VSD	Note: Normal patent foramen ovale may be seen between atria Isolated finding or part of a complex or syndrome
Enlarged right atrium apical displacement of with tricuspid valve Septal defects, tetralogy of Fallot, coarctation of aorta may be noted Hydrops (if condition is severe)	Uterus may measure large for dates	Ebstein anomaly	Associated with micrognathia, cleft lip/palate, agenesis of left kidney, megacolon, and undescended testes

continued

Second and Third Trimester Fetal Thorax and Heart—*cont'd*

Sonographic Finding(s)	Clinical Presentation	Differential Diagnosis	Next Step
All chambers of heart appear enlarged Cardiac muscle may appear thin Hydrops	Asymptomatic	Cardiomyopathy Pseudocardiomegaly (small thorax) Outflow tract obstruction Ebstein's anomaly	This finding may be an isolated finding or may be part of a complex or syndrome
Heart is on right side of thorax	Asymptomatic	Dextrocardia	Isolated finding or may be part of a complex or syndrome Heart may be displaced to right by pathologic condition in left thorax

Unable to visualize crossing of great vessels in short-axis view; outflow tracts are parallel VSD	Asymptomatic	Transposition of great arteries Double outlet right ventricle Tetralogy of Fallot	Rarely associated with aneuploidy
Heart is outside thorax or displaced into fetal abdomen	Asymptomatic	Ectopia cordis	Isolated finding or associated with limb–body wall complex, pentalogy of Cantrell
Mass(es) within heart Hydrops Cardiac arrhythmia may be noted	Uterus may measure large for dates	Rhabdomyoma Teratoma Hemangioma Fibroma Hypertrophic cardiomyopathy (wall thickening)	Do not confuse with normal papillary muscle (brightly echogenic) May regress in utero Fetal death may occur

continued

Second and Third Trimester Fetal Thorax and Heart—*cont'd*

Sonographic Finding(s)	Clinical Presentation	Differential Diagnosis	Next Step
Solid or cystic mass within lung Cystic type may be microcystic (echogenic) or macrocystic (1 or more cysts 5.0 mm or greater) Hydrops	Asymptomatic	CAM Pulmonary sequestration Diaphragmatic hernia Bronchogenic cyst	Incidental finding Stable or may regress in utero May lead to fetal death Solid mass with color Doppler evidence of feeding vessel and pleural effusion is more likely pulmonary sequestration

Second and Third Trimester Fetal GI System

Sonographic Finding(s)	Clinical Presentation	Differential Diagnosis	Next Step
Polyhydramnios and lack of visualization or very small size of stomach Polyhydramnios may be mild or massive	Uterus may measure large for dates	Esophageal atresia TE fistula Diaphragmatic hernia Abnormal swallowing CNS anomaly	Isolated finding or may be part of a complex or syndrome: VACTERL
Fluid surrounds abdominal organs Amount of fluid may be small to large	Uterus may measure large for dates	Fetal ascites	Isolated finding or may be associated with fetal hydrops
Fetal stomach located in left thorax; fetal heart may be displaced to right Polyhydramnios	Uterus may measure large for dates	Diaphragmatic hernia CAM	Associated with abnormal cardiac axis, pulmonary hypoplasia; CNS, cardiac, renal and spinal anomalies; trisomy 13, 18, 21 *continued*

Second and Third Trimester Fetal GI System—*cont'd*

Sonographic Finding(s)	Clinical Presentation	Differential Diagnosis	Next Step
Two or more cystic structures are noted in fetal abdomen A connection between the stomach and the adjacent cystic structure may be noted Amniotic fluid level may be normal to mild polyhydramnios	Uterus may measure large for dates	Duodenal atresia Jejunal atresia	Associated with trisomy 21, skeletal, cardiac, and other GI abnormalities
Additional cystic structure visualized adjacent to gallbladder is noted	Asymptomatic	Choledochal cyst Liver cyst Gallbladder duplication Mesenteric cyst Ovarian cyst	Confirm position of gallbladder
Floating structures are noted adjacent to right	Uterus may measure small for dates, especially	Gastroschisis Omphalocele	This finding is not generally associated with the

of the umbilical cord; normal umbilical cord insertion into fetal abdomen not seen May demonstrate thin (early) to thick (late) walls May demonstrate as fluid-filled structures	abdominal circumference Labs: elevated MSAFP	Limb–body wall complex	presence of other fetal anomalies Oligohydramnios may be present
Umbilical cord inserts into a mass rather than the fetal abdomen The mass most likely contains solid tissue (liver) but may contain bowel loops The mass may be small to large	Uterus measures large for dates Labs: elevated MSAFP	Omphalocele Gastroschisis Umbilical hernia	Isolated finding or may be part of a complex or syndrome: Beckwith-Wiedemann, pentalogy of Cantrell

continued

Second and Third Trimester Fetal GI System—*cont'd*

Sonographic Finding(s)	Clinical Presentation	Differential Diagnosis	Next Step
Cystic structure noted in the abdomen	Asymptomatic	Duplication cyst/ovarian cyst Choledochal cyst Dilated bowel	May be an isolated finding
Echogenic bowel; ≥liver, <bone Echogenicities in abdomen IGUR Hydrops	Uterus may measure small or large for dates	Hyperechoic bowel Meconium ileus/peritonitis Cystic fibrosis	Isolated finding or associated with trisomy 21, CMV Focal echogenicity more pathologic than diffuse echogenic bowel

Second and Third Trimester Fetal Urinary System

Sonographic Finding(s)	Clinical Presentation	Differential Diagnosis	Next Step
Dilated renal pelvis (AP diameter >2.0 cm) Dilated calyces may/may not be seen Renal parenchyma may appear thin Dilated ureters may/may not be seen If bilateral, oligohydramnios is likely Dilated urinary bladder may/may not be seen	Uterus may measure small for dates	Hydronephrosis Idiopathic pyelectasis MCDK	"Cysts" connect to central large "cyst" Associated with UPJ obstruction; soft marker for trisomy 21

continued

Second and Third Trimester Fetal Urinary System—*cont'd*

Sonographic Finding(s)	Clinical Presentation	Differential Diagnosis	Next Step
Kidneys are enlarged and may demonstrate some to significantly increased echogenicity No urinary bladder is noted Oligohydramnios is noted	Uterus may measure small for dates	ARPKD	This finding is always bilateral and is one of the presentations of Potter's syndrome (type II)
Kidney appears very small or unable to find kidney; adrenal gland is prominent and elongated If unilateral, contralateral kidney may be larger than normal and the urinary bladder is seen If bilateral, urinary bladder will not be seen and oligohydramnios is noted	Uterus measures small for dates	Renal agenesis	Isolated finding or may be part of a complex or syndrome (Potter's syndrome type II)

Multiple cysts of different sizes noted in area of renal fossa	Uterus may measure small for dates	Multicystic kidney	Isolated finding or associated with Potter's syndrome type II if bilateral
Solid mass within kidney; may seem "superior" to kidney Contralateral kidney may be larger than normal Urinary bladder is seen	Asymptomatic	Wilms' tumor (nephroblastoma) Mesoblastic nephroma Neuroblastoma Adrenal hemorrhage	Neuroblastoma and adrenal hemorrhage displace kidney
Inferior poles of kidneys appear closer to midline (abnormal lie of kidneys) with a small amount of solid tissue connecting poles May occur at superior poles	Uterus may measure large for dates if hydrops is present	Horseshoe kidney	Isolated finding or may be part of a complex or syndrome: trisomy 13, 18; Turner's syndrome

continued

Second and Third Trimester Fetal Urinary System—*cont'd*

Sonographic Finding(s)	Clinical Presentation	Differential Diagnosis	Next Step
Dilated tubular structures posterior to bowel Hydronephrosis may/may not be seen Urinary bladder may/may not be seen Oligohydramnios	Uterus may measure small for dates	Megaureter Urethral atresia Prune-belly syndrome Megacystis	Isolated finding or associated with posterior urethral valves
Urinary bladder is seen outside fetal abdomen/pelvis Bladder is not seen after scanning for >30 minutes Umbilical arteries are demonstrated with color Doppler imaging	Uterus may measure small for dates Labs: elevated MSAFP	Bladder exstrophy Cloacal exstrophy	Associated with reproductive tract abnormalities Not associated with pregnancy complications

Fetal anatomy difficult to visualize; large pocket of fluid extends from fetal pelvis to abdomen Hydronephrosis with/without hydroureter Oligohydramnios	Uterus may measure large or small for dates	Posterior urethral valves	The large pocket of fluid is not amniotic fluid; it is the fetal urinary bladder that is massively distended
Female fetus demonstrates oval fluid-filled area in pelvis/lower abdomen	Asymptomatic	Hydrocolpos	This finding is not associated with other anomalies but may mimic other abdominal cysts or the urinary bladder

Second and Third Trimester Fetal Spine and Skeleton

Sonographic Finding(s)	Clinical Presentation	Differential Diagnosis	Next Step
Fetal spine demonstrates splaying of posterior elements ("U" or "V" shape in transverse axis) Polyhydramnios Ventriculomegaly, Chiari type II malformation, club foot, cleft lip/palate, cephalocele, hypotelorism, heart defects, and GU anomalies may be noted Meningocele or meningomyelocele may be noted	Asymptomatic Maternal diabetes Folic acid deficiency History of exposure to teratogens or maternal hyperthermia Labs: elevated AFP if defect is open	Spina bifida (general term for lack of closure of neural tube) May present as Rachischisis Meningocele Meningomyelocele	Most commonly located in caudal sections of spine May be sporadic or associated with genetic anomalies

Fetal spine demonstrates splaying of posterior elements ("U" or "V" shape in transverse axis) without skin covering defect

A pouch may be noted protruding from spine

Ventriculomegaly, Chiari type II malformation, clubfoot, cleft lip/palate, cephalocele, hypotelorism, heart defects, and GU anomalies may be noted

Asymptomatic
Maternal diabetes
Folic acid deficiency
History of exposure to teratogens or maternal hyperthermia
Labs: elevated AFP, MSAFP, ACE

Spinal rachischisis
Meningocele
Meningomyelocele (myelomeningocele)

Demonstrate defect in coronal and transverse
Demonstrate presence of meninges and cord within protruding pouch
Establish level of defect
IUGR may be present

continued

Second and Third Trimester Fetal Spine and Skeleton—*cont'd*

Sonographic Finding(s)	Clinical Presentation	Differential Diagnosis	Next Step
Complex mass extending from sacrum; calcifications may be noted Color Doppler imaging demonstrates hypervascularity of mass Placentomegaly Polyhydramnios	Uterus measures large for dates Labs: elevated AFP if open neural tube defect is present	Sacrococcygeal teratoma	More common in females Hydronephrosis may be present Hydrops may develop
Foot or hand consistently at abnormal axis to leg or arm Additional fetal anomalies may or may not be noted May be due to postural restriction May be bilateral	Asymptomatic Labs: elevated AFP if open neural tube defect is present	Clubfoot/club hand	Clubfoot may be sporadic or associated with syndromes and genetic anomalies Club hand is associated with syndromes or genetic anomalies including trisomies and VATER

Foot has convex shape; commonly bilateral	Asymptomatic Labs: elevated AFP if open neural tube defect is present	Rocker-bottom foot	Associated with trisomy 13, 18
Shortening of arms and legs (rhizomelia or micromelia) Bowed femurs Large, asymmetric head; may demonstrate with frontal bossing (prominent forehead) Hypertelorism Narrow thorax with protuberant abdomen Flattened vertebral bodies Polyhydramnios, hydrocephalus, and hydrops may be noted	Uterus may measure large for dates	Thanatophoric dysplasia Achondrogenesis Achondroplasia Camptomelic dysplasia	Lethal skeletal dysplasia: small thorax leads to pulmonary hypoplasia

continued

Second and Third Trimester Fetal Spine and Skeleton—*cont'd*

Sonographic Finding(s)	Clinical Presentation	Differential Diagnosis	Next Step
Extremities are oddly positioned Polyhydramnios Small thorax and umbilical cord IUGR may be present	Uterus measures large for dates Decreased fetal movements	Arthrogryposis (joint contractures) Trisomy 18	Description of finding, not a diagnosis Associated with agenesis of the corpus callosum, lissencephaly, Dandy-Walker malformation, trisomy 18

Limbs appear short
Limbs 2 standard deviations below mean
	Uterus may measure large for dates because of polyhydramnios	Short-limb dysplasia:
		  Rhizomelia (proximal extremities)
		  Mesomelia (distal extremities)
		  Micromelia (proximal and distal extremities)
			Feature of thanatophoric dysplasia, camptomelic dysplasia, osteogenesis imperfecta type II, and nonlethal skeletal dysplasias

Large head with bulging forehead (frontal bossing) Flat nasal bridge Gap between third and fourth fingers Shortened femurs in third trimester (abnormal HC/FL ratio) Polyhydramnios may be noted	Uterus may measure large for dates if polyhydramnios is present	Achondroplasia Osteogenesis imperfecta Thanatophoric dysplasia	Heterozygous form is most common nonlethal skeletal dysplasia Homozygous is lethal form
Large head with normal or decreased ossification; lack of ossification of spine Micrognathia Shortened limbs, small thorax, large abdomen Hydrops	Uterus measures large for dates	Achondrogenesis (failure of ossification process) Osteogenesis imperfecta Hypophosphatasia	Lethal skeletal dysplasia May be genetic or sporadic occurrence

continued

Second and Third Trimester Fetal Spine and Skeleton—*cont'd*

Sonographic Finding(s)	Clinical Presentation	Differential Diagnosis	Next Step
Extremities are short with evidence of angulation or fractures; bones may appear "bumpy" from callus formation Small thorax; rib fractures Brain is easily seen because of poor ossification of skull Possible polyhydramnios	Uterus may be large for dates because of polyhydramnios	Osteogenesis imperfecta (sonographic appearances vary with type) Hypophosphatasia Achondrogenesis Camptomelic dysplasia	May be autosomal recessive or dominant Types I and IV: not seen in utero Type II: severe form, lethal Type III: multiple fractures Transducer pressure may deform skull
Short or absent radius Club hand Absent thumb	History of exposure to teratogens: thalidomide, cocaine, evaporate, and vitamin A Uterus may measure small for dates if oligohydramnios is present	Radial ray aphasia/hypoplasia Osteogenesis imperfecta	Associated with VACTERL, trisomy 18, and Holt-Oram syndrome (cardiac anomalies)

Extra digits on hands or feet Digits may be small, wide, or abnormally located	Asymptomatic	Polydactyly	Associated with numerous conditions: Trisomy 13 Meckel-Gruber syndrome Ellis-van Creveld syndrome Smith-Lemi-Opitz syndrome Confirm that hands/feet are separate when documenting this finding

Second and Third Trimester Fetal Syndromes

Sonographic Finding(s)	Clinical Presentation	Differential Diagnosis	Next Step
Nuchal translucency measurement >3.0 mm between 9 and 13 weeks' gestation (45.0 mm–84.0 mm CRL)	Asymptomatic Screening exam: advanced maternal age Labs: abnormal PAPP-A, triple or quadruple screen	Increased nuchal translucency	Accuracy of measurement is critical Associated with numerous genetic and nongenetic abnormalities/defects and cardiac defects
Increased nuchal translucency Cardiac defects, duodenal atresia, nuchal skin thickening, short femurs, echogenic bowel, ventriculomegaly, echogenic intracardiac focus, renal pelvicectasis, clinodactyly, sandal gap foot may be noted in second-trimester fetus	Asymptomatic Advanced maternal age Labs: low AFP, elevated β-hCG, low estriol, high inhibin A protein (abnormal quadruple screen)	Trisomy 21 (Down syndrome) Isolated anomalies not related to trisomy 21	Combination of abnormal nuchal translucency and quadruple screen improves detection rate for trisomy 21 Presence of multiple "soft" ultrasound markers increases likelihood of trisomy 21 Nuchal fold thickness not useful after 22 weeks' gestation

IUGR, cardiac defects, cystic hygroma, bowel-containing omphalocele, "strawberry"-shaped head, choroid plexus cysts, two-vessel umbilical cord, clenched hands with overlapped index finger, abnormal feet, hypertelorism, micrognatia, spina bifida	Asymptomatic Uterus may measure large for dates if polyhydramnios is present Advanced maternal age Labs: abnormal triple screen	Trisomy 18 (Edwards syndrome) Isolated anomalies not related to trisomy 18 Triploidy	If choroid plexus cyst is found, carefully check hands and heart (VSD, ASD, or dextrocardia) Polyhydramnios, cleft lip/palate, diaphragmatic hernia, and cerebellar hypoplasia may also be noted
Holoprosencephaly, agenesis of corpus callosum, cerebellar anomaly, cleft lip/palate, cyclopia/hypotelorism, proboscis, clenched hands, polydactyly, clubfeet, IUGR	Asymptomatic Uterus may measure large for dates if polyhydramnios is present Advanced maternal age Labs: low AFP	Trisomy 13 (Patau syndrome) Meckel-Gruber syndrome Holoprosencephaly (isolated finding)	Suspect brain anomaly if facial anomaly is seen Intracardiac echogenic focus, single umbilical artery, increased nuchal translucency or fold, and echogenic bowel may be seen

continued

Second and Third Trimester Fetal Syndromes—*cont'd*

Sonographic Finding(s)	Clinical Presentation	Differential Diagnosis	Next Step
Asymmetric, random, bizarre slash defects: facial clefts, cephaloceles, anencephaly, amputation of an extremity Constriction of an extremity with edema Thorax and abdominal wall defects Oligohydramnios may be noted	Uterus may measure small for dates	Amniotic band syndrome (disruption of amnion with entrapment of fetal anatomy) Limb–body all complex Amniotic sheets Chorioamniotic separation	May present as thin band(s) floating in amniotic fluid May see fetus entangled in a band Amniotic sheets and chorioamniotic separation do not entrap fetus
Bilateral large echogenic kidneys; large cysts may be present Urinary bladder not seen	Uterus measures small for dates Labs: elevated AFP if encephalocele is present	Meckel-Gruber syndrome Trisomy 13 ARPKD MCDK	Significant overlap with findings of trisomy 13 Renal appearance is often variable; large kidneys can increase abdominal circumference

Oligohydramnios Encephalocele Polydactyly Cleft lip/palate, micrognathia Cardiac septal defect Small thorax		Encephalocele (isolated finding)	
Ectopia cordis with omphalocele Diaphragmatic hernia Pleural or pericardial effusion	Asymptomatic	Pentalogy of Cantrell Isolated ectopia cordis Isolated omphalocele Limb–body wall complex Amniotic band syndrome	Associated with cardiac anomalies, cleft lip/palate, encephalocele, trisomies 13 and 18, Turner's syndrome, and cystic hygroma
Oligohydramnios Small thorax Unable to detect urinary bladder	Uterus measures small for dates Decreased fetal movements	Potter's syndrome/sequence PROM Severe IUGR	Lack of urine production can be related to bladder exstrophy or rupture Associated with pulmonary hypoplasia

continued

Second and Third Trimester Fetal Syndromes—*cont'd*

Sonographic Finding(s)	Clinical Presentation	Differential Diagnosis	Next Step
Bilateral renal agenesis (elongated and prominent adrenal glands) *or* Bilateral MCDK *or* ARPKD			
Ventriculomegaly Syndactyly Severe asymmetric IUGR Large cystic placenta (molar placenta); bilateral theca lutein cysts Oligohydramnios Single umbilical artery Omphalocele	Vaginal bleeding Labs: paternal source demonstrates elevated β-hCG, AFP, inhibin A; decreased PAPP-A Maternal source demonstrates decreased quadruple screen	Triploidy Hydatidiform mole with coexistent fetus Fetal death with molar degeneration of the placenta Placental lakes Pseudomole Trisomies 18, 13	Multiple CNS, face/neck, cardiac, GU anomalies may be noted Usually results in pregnancy loss before 20 weeks Lethal

Cystic hygroma	Uterus may measure large or small for dates (oligohydramnios related to IUGR)	Turner syndrome (45,X)	Use high gain settings to demonstrate thin septations in cystic hygroma
Hydrops		Noonan syndrome	
Symmetric IUGR		Trisomy 21	
Horseshoe kidneys			Cystic hygroma can mimic amniotic fluid
Mild rhizomelia	Labs: decreased quadruple screen; elevated β-hCG and inhibin A if hydrops is present		
Normal female genitalia			Coarctation of the aorta may be seen

Second and Third Trimester Multiple Gestation

Sonographic Finding(s)	Clinical Presentation	Differential Diagnosis	Next Step
Thick membrane separates fetuses	Uterus measures large for dates	DZ:DC/DA twins	Membranes are thicker than MC/DA twins
Chorionic "peak" or "λ" sign is noted (presence of placental tissue between membranes) indicating the presence of adjacent placentas	Increased nausea and vomiting is possible	MZ:DC/DA twins (if fetuses are same sex)	Risk of preterm delivery is greater than for singleton pregnancy
Placentas may be widely separated	Labs: increase in β-hCG and AFP		Associated with development of maternal hypertension, preeclampsia, and hemorrhage (placenta previa, placental abruption)
Fetuses are same (monozygotic) or opposite sex (dizygotic)			Some increased risk of IUGR and fetal anomalies

Single placenta noted Lack of chorionic "peak" or "λ" sign Thin membrane between fetuses Fetuses same sex Discordant growth may be present Discordant amniotic fluid volume may be noted	Uterus measures large for dates Increased nausea and vomiting is possible Labs: increase in β-hCG and AFP	MC/DA twins	Identify placental cord insertion sites Increased risk of fetal CNS and cardiac anomalies and vasa previa Associated with IUGR, TTTS, TRAP, and TES At risk for loss of one or both fetuses
Single placenta noted Unable to identify membrane between fetuses Fetuses same sex Umbilical cords appear entangled or fused Discordant growth may be present	Uterus measures large for dates Increased nausea and vomiting is possible Labs: increase in β-hCG and AFP	MC/MA twins Conjoined twins DA twins with absent membrane	High risk of pregnancy loss Associated with lethal fetal anomalies, TTTS, locking twins

continued

Second and Third Trimester Multiple Gestation—*cont'd*

Sonographic Finding(s)	Clinical Presentation	Differential Diagnosis	Next Step
Single placenta noted Unable to demonstrate fetuses separately; fusion of variable degree Fetuses have different heart rates	Uterus measures large for dates Increased nausea and vomiting is possible History of long-term oral contraceptive use Labs: increase in β-hCG, AFP	Conjoined twins MA twins Locking twins TRAP	Increased risk of preterm delivery and stillborn delivery Must demonstrate contiguous skin covering
MC/DA twins with asymmetric fluid and growth One fetus in an oligohydramniotic sac (closely applied membrane; "stuck" twin) Polyhydramnios Abnormal umbilical artery flow	Uterus may measure large for dates Labs: increase in β-hCG and AFP	TTTS	Associated with shared placenta with shunting vessels, cardiac defects, hydrops in recipient twin, and echogenic bowel in donor twin Risk for death of one or both fetuses

Unable to detect fetal heart motion
Subcutaneous edema
Overlapping skull sutures (Spaulding's sign)
Unnatural fetal position
Loss of definition of structures in abdomen; gas in fetal abdomen (Robert's sign)
Oligohydramnios may be noted

Decreased fetal movements
Unable to hear fetal heart tones
Vaginal bleeding with cramping
Decreased fundal height
Labs: negative β-hCG

Fetal death
Severe oligohydramnios limits fetal movement
Maternal obesity limits physical and ultrasound exam (normal fetus)

Maternal pulse may be mistaken for fetal movement
Serial sonograms may be needed
Associated with maternal hypertension, diabetes; infection; fetal anomalies; PROM

Uterus, Placenta, Umbilical Cord, and Fluid

Sonographic Finding(s)	Clinical Presentation	Differential Diagnosis	Next Step
Hypoechoic to hyperechoic rounded structure in uterine wall; single or multiple Does not change in size during sonogram May distort contour of uterus May distort uterine cavity	Asymptomatic *or* Pregnancy is large for dates by palpation Possible pain, contractions, vaginal bleeding	Leiomyoma (fibroid) Uterine contraction Placenta previa	Document location and size; may enlarge during pregnancy Evaluate location relative to placenta and cervical os May cause malposition of uterus or fetus or spontaneous abortion
Cystic mass in maternal adnexa	Asymptomatic *or* Pelvic pain/discomfort	Persistent corpus luteum cyst Dermoid Dilated ureter Mucinous/serous cystadenoma Paraovarian cyst	A corpus luteum cyst should regress by 15 weeks' gestation

| Single or multiple hypoechoic areas or lesions noted within the placenta or may be subchorionic
Swirling blood may be seen with 2D imaging | Asymptomatic
Labs: elevated AFP may be noted | Placental lakes
Venous lakes
Intervillous thrombus
Fibrin deposits
Chorioangioma
Gestational trophoblastic disease
Placental abruption | Placental lakes may change size during exam because of uterine contractions
Increased risk of placental insufficiency
Increase gain settings to visualize swirling blood (color Doppler imaging not helpful) |
| Anechoic tubular structures posterior to placenta, between basal plate and myometrium | Asymptomatic | Prominent marginal veins (retroplacental complex)
Retroplacental hemorrhage | Use color Doppler imaging to confirm blood flow within structures |

continued

Uterus, Placenta, Umbilical Cord, and Fluid—cont'd

Sonographic Finding(s)	Clinical Presentation	Differential Diagnosis	Next Step
Cervix length is shorter than normal with EV or transperineal imaging (length <25.0 mm at or before 24 weeks' gestation) Funneling appearance of internal os (>50% of cervical length) Bulging membranes may be noted	Asymptomatic History of preterm delivery, multiple gestation, or cervical surgery (cone, LEEP, etc.) Possible vaginal bleeding or leakage of amniotic fluid	Incompetent cervix Overly distended maternal urinary bladder; lower uterine contraction (either may mimic cervical funneling or obscure shortened cervix)	Evaluate cervix immediately after patient is supine If risk factors are present or cervix appears short, apply fundal pressure; document length of cervix with/without fundal pressure Use transperineal technique if bleeding, leakage of fluid, or cervical dilation are noted
Edge of the placenta is noted very near internal cervical os	Asymptomatic	Low-lying placenta	False positive because of Braxton-Hicks contraction or fibroid in lower uterine segment

Fetus is completely surrounded by and is free floating in amniotic fluid AFI >25.0 cm Single pocket >8.0 cm Placenta may appear thinned	Uterus measures large for dates Maternal diabetes	Polyhydramnios	Associated with esophageal or duodenal atresia, skeletal and CNS anomalies, fetal hydrops
Visualization of fetal anatomy is limited or impossible Little or no amniotic fluid noted AFI <5.0 cm Single pocket <2.0 cm	Uterus measures small for dates Loss or leaking of amniotic fluid (PROM) Known polyhydramnios	Oligohydramnios	Associated with renal agenesis and urinary bladder obstruction. May be the result of PROM
Single umbilical artery and vein are noted by 2D and color Doppler imaging	Asymptomatic	Two-vessel cord/single umbilical artery	Associated with several fetal anomalies

continued

Uterus, Placenta, Umbilical Cord, and Fluid—*cont'd*

Sonographic Finding(s)	Clinical Presentation	Differential Diagnosis	Next Step

All or part of placenta covers internal os of cervix
Fetal head is >1.5 cm from sacrum with posterior placenta
	Painless vaginal bleeding	Placenta previa types:
		  Marginal
		  Partial
		  Complete
			Use translabial or EV imaging to demonstrate placental relationship to cervix

Placental thickness is >4.0 cm throughout	Uterus may measure large for dates	Placentomegaly Placental abruption (abruptio placentae) Leiomyoma Gestational trophoblastic disease	More common with lateral placenta Associated with macrosomia, maternal diabetes, hydrops, molar pregnancy
Placental edge is displaced away from uterine wall Hematoma noted at edge of placenta	Vaginal bleeding with/without pain History of previous placental abruption	Marginal placental abruption	Most common type of abruption Large abruption may affect fetal well-being

Central detachment of placenta from uterine wall May at first appear as focal thickening of placenta; sonographic appearance of hematoma changes with time	Vaginal bleeding with/without pain Pain can be severe with massive hemorrhage Uterus may become rigid and "board-like"	Retroplacental abruption Leiomyoma Braxton-Hicks contraction Chorioangioma	Significant finding Large hemorrhage may be life threatening; small bleeding episode may be "silent"
Echogenic linear structures around periphery of cervix	History of incompetent cervix	Cervical cerclage (sutures to maintain a closed cervix)	Most common technique is the purse-string method
Complex or solid mass in the maternal adnexa	Asymptomatic *or* Pelvic pain/discomfort	Dermoid Endometrioma Pelvic kidney Nongravid horn of bicornuate uterus Fecal-filled colon Myometrial contraction	If myometrial contraction (Braxton-Hicks contraction) is suspected, rescan in a few minutes

continued

Uterus, Placenta, Umbilical Cord, and Fluid—*cont'd*

Sonographic Finding(s)	Clinical Presentation	Differential Diagnosis	Next Step
Hypoechoic mass within placenta often near the cord insertion Color Doppler imaging demonstrates flow within the mass	Asymptomatic *or* Uterus large for dates because of polyhydramnios Labs: elevated AFP with large chorioangioma	Chorioangioma Venous lakes Intervillous thrombi Placental abruption (preplacental) Leiomyoma Teratoma Gestational trophoblastic disease	Use of color Doppler imaging essential for diagnosis 3D imaging may be useful If large, fetus may have hydrops
In a singleton pregnancy, placenta is noted in two or more separate locations IUGR may be noted	Asymptomatic Vaginal bleeding	Succenturiate placenta (accessory placenta) Placental abruption Braxton-Hicks contraction	Connecting membrane may cross internal cervical os Vasa previa and velamentous cord insertion may be present Increased risk for cord rupture and retained placenta

Umbilical cord is noted between fetal presenting part and cervix at term May be transient finding throughout pregnancy	Asymptomatic	Vasa previa	Associated with succenturiate placenta and velamentous cord insertion into placenta

Unable to visualize hypoechoic subplacental zone
Placenta previa
Thinned myometrium or placenta attached to bladder wall may be noted (mass effect in bladder)
	Heavy bleeding during labor
	History of previous cesarean section deliveries
	Advanced maternal age
		Placenta:
		  Accreta
		  Increta
		  Percreta
		Placental previa
		Gestational trophoblastic disease
			In cases of placenta percreta, the chorionic villi may invade maternal bladder wall

continued

Uterus, Placenta, Umbilical Cord, and Fluid—*cont'd*

Sonographic Finding(s)	Clinical Presentation	Differential Diagnosis	Next Step
Elevated placental margins Peripheral echogenic rim ("shelf")	Possible vaginal bleeding	Circumvallate placenta Uterine synechia (amniotic sheets) Amniotic bands Septate uterus	Associated with IUGR, PROM, or preterm labor and delivery Often an incidental finding
Umbilical cord inserts within 2.0 cm of placental edge noted with 2D and color Doppler imaging Branching vessels noted on placental surface	Asymptomatic	Battledore placenta Velamentous cord insertion Adjacent cord	Increased incidence with MC twins Velamentous cord may develop
Umbilical cord inserts into membranes noted with 2D and color Doppler	Asymptomatic until delivery	Velamentous cord insertion Battledore placenta Marginal placental previa	Associated with abnormal placentation and MC twins

Large soft tissue mass within uterus without evidence of fetus or fetal parts Placenta fills uterus and demonstrates cystic change Bilateral theca lutein cysts	Uterus is large for dates Unable to discern fetal heart tones Vaginal bleeding Hyperemesis Preeclampsia Labs: elevated serum β-hCG (>100,000 mIU/ml)	Gestational trophoblastic disease (mole) Hydatidiform Invasive mole (chorioadenoma destruens) Choriocarcinoma	Invasive mole may penetrate uterine wall Metastatic spread to liver, lung, and brain with choriocarcinoma
Large soft tissue mass within uterus with cystic changes Presence of small fetus or fetal parts Bilateral theca lutein cysts	Large for dates Unable to discern fetal heart tones Vaginal bleeding (may be heavy) Hyperemesis Preeclampsia Labs: elevated serum β-hCG (>100,000 mIU/ml)	Partial/incomplete mole Hydropic degeneration of placenta	Associated with triploid fetus

continued

Uterus, Placenta, Umbilical Cord, and Fluid—*cont'd*

Sonographic Finding(s)	Clinical Presentation	Differential Diagnosis	Next Step
Molar placenta with normal placenta and fetus	Uterus is large for dates Vaginal bleeding (may be heavy) Passage of grape-like tissue Hyperemesis Preeclampsia Labs: elevated serum β-hCG (>100,000 mIU/ml)	Coexistent mole (molar degeneration of one gestation of a twin pregnancy)	Rare finding Coexisting fetus and placenta will appear normal

PEDIATRICS

Chapter 16 Pediatric Studies

Patient Preparation

- Fasting time is not necessary or shorter for the pediatric age groups. No preparation for urinary examinations is required, but the bladder should not be emptied immediately before the examination. Pelvic sonograms in children should only require that the child not void immediately before the examination.

- Examining babies and small children requires that distractions are used to obtain cooperation during the examination. A parent should be in the room with the child. The examination should be explained to the parent or to the older child; demonstrate putting the transducer on your skin to show that the examination will not hurt.

- Neonates should be kept as warm as possible during the examination; warm gel should always be used, an external warming lamp may be used, and time spent scanning should be kept to a minimum. The neonate should be disturbed as little as possible.

- Neurosonograms require that the anterior fontanelle is accessible (intravenous needle must be removed).

Equipment and Technical Factors

- High-frequency transducers are commonly used for babies and small children. A linear array is used for pylorus and hip studies. A small footprint, high-frequency annular array, or sector transducer is used for neurosonograms of neonates; infants and older babies may require a lower-frequency transducer.

- Multiple focal zones may be used for a neurosonogram.

- Color Doppler imaging can be used to distinguish vascular from nonvascular structures and to identify vessels adjacent to the organ/structure of interest.

- MI/TI settings should be kept very low.
- Transducer covers should be used in cases of suspected infection.

Imaging Protocol

- Minimum documentation images for all examinations should include longitudinal and transverse axes images. Breathing techniques can be used for older children.

Minimum documentation images for the pylorus

- Longitudinal and transverse axes images with measurement of the length and wall thickness of the pylorus should be obtained. Images demonstrating fluid in the antrum of the stomach with or without passage of the fluid through the pylorus should be obtained. The patient may be placed supine or in a right oblique or decubitus position.

Minimum documentation images for the neurosonogram

- Specific positioning of the head is not as critical as is access to the anterior fontanelle. The anterior fontanelle coronal and modified coronal planes (C1–C7) are used to demonstrate the frontal lobes through the occipital lobes and the sagittal and parasagittal planes (ML-Sag 3–4) to demonstrate the midline structures through the far lateral aspect of the brain.
- Sagittal and parasagittal imaging should display the anterior portion of the brain toward the left of the screen and the posterior portion to the right. The coronal and modified coronal images, which display the right side of the brain, are on the left side of the screen.
- Other fontanelles may be used for imaging, if needed, but will not result in the above standard images.

Minimum documentation images for the dynamic infant hip examination

- Coronal and transverse images of the acetabulum and femoral head and neck with the hip in neutral position at rest and in flexion should be obtained. With hip flexion, the femur is abducted, adducted and stress maneuvers are done.
- Examination without abduction, adduction, and stress maneuvers may be done with the infant in a Pavlik harness.

Measurements

CBD

- <1.0 mm neonate
- <2.0 mm infant less than 2 years of age
- <4.0 mm child between 2 and 12 years of age
- <5.0 mm adolescent

Kidneys

- Size varies with age. In older children, kidney size can also be related to the height and weight of the child if the kidneys are small or large for age.

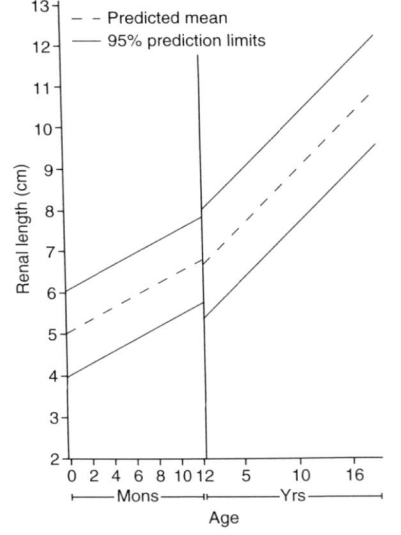

Normal renal length versus age. (From Rumack CM, Wilson SR, Charboneau WJ et al: *Diagnostic ultrasound*, ed 3, vol 2, 2005, St. Louis, Mosby/Elsevier.)

Pylorus

- <3.5 mm wall thickness
- <17.0 mm in length

Uterus (Premenarchal)

- Length: 3.3–5.4 cm (cervix: 3.0 cm)
- Width: 0.7–1.6 cm
- Depth (AP): 0.7–1.6 cm
- Neonate: Uterine fundus larger than in a child because of maternal hormone stimulus

Ovarian volume

- 0.523 (L × W × D)
- Premenarchal: 3.0 cm^3

Neurosonogram (neonate)

- Oblique diameter of ventricle body: <3.0 mm
- Width of third ventricle in coronal view: <2.0 mm

Pediatric Studies

Sonographic Finding(s)	Clinical Presentation	Differential Diagnosis	Next Step

Pyloric wall is thickened and pylorus is elongated
  Thickness of wall: >4.0 mm
  Length: >17.0 mm
"Beaking" sign of fluid in antrum
	Usually a first-born infant male, 4–6 weeks of age
	Projectile vomiting
	Failure to thrive (FTT)
		Hypertrophic pyloric stenosis	Evaluate pylorus for spasm, passage of fluid

In a newborn/infant/child, a kidney is absent in renal fossa, the ipsilateral adrenal is elongated, and renal arteries cannot be demonstrated with color Doppler imaging Ipsilateral ectopic kidney is not identified	Suspected anomaly from prenatal sonogram	Unilateral renal agenesis	Associated with reproductive system anomalies Contralateral kidney will be normal sized at birth but will demonstrate compensatory hypertrophy between 6–12 months of age

Kidney has a "lumpy" appearance	Asymptomatic	Fetal lobulation	Normal feature of kidney development in utero that may persist into adulthood
Triangular echogenic focus noted between the mid and upper sections of kidney	Asymptomatic	Junctional parenchymal defect	May also be seen with an interrenicular septum Remnant of fetal renal lobes
Cortical tissue is noted between areas of echogenic renal pelvis Kidney may be normal or somewhat larger in size May be noted bilaterally	Asymptomatic	Bifid renal pelvis	Mildest form of kidney duplication Renal pelvis is singular at the renal hilum

continued

Pediatric Studies—*cont'd*

Sonographic Finding(s)	Clinical Presentation	Differential Diagnosis	Next Step
Duplication of renal collecting system with duplication of proximal ureters Ureters may rejoin distal to kidney and proximal to bladder Kidney is usually larger than normal May be noted bilaterally	Asymptomatic	Partial duplication Duplex collecting system	Reproductive anomalies may be present
Duplication of renal collecting system and ureters Ureters enter bladder through separate orifices Hydronephrosis of the superior pole collecting system with/without hydroureter may be noted May be noted bilaterally	History of urinary tract infections	Complete duplication	Ureterocele may be noted as superior pole ureter inserts abnormally Echogenic dysplastic parenchyma may develop in upper pole of kidney

Hydronephrosis in an infant or child Dilated calyces connect with dilated renal pelvis May be unilateral or bilateral	Abnormal prenatal sonogram Child: pain, hematuria, urinary tract infection, increased fluid intake	UPJ obstruction	Most common cause of hydronephrosis in children If bilateral, renal function may be affected
Large, dilated, tortuous ureter(s) that tapers distally (at bladder)	Obstructive and reflux have symptoms and abnormal lab values	Megaureter	Associated with UVJ obstruction or urinary reflux (neurogenic bladder, ectopic ureterocele, posterior urethral valves)
Cystic structure noted in urinary bladder	Asymptomatic	Ureterocele Ectopic ureterocele	May be an incidental finding Ectopic ureterocele is associated with complete duplication of renal collecting system (abnormal insertion of ureter) or urinary obstruction (children) *continued*

Pediatric Studies—*cont'd*

Sonographic Finding(s)	Clinical Presentation	Differential Diagnosis	Next Step
Male neonate with dilated, thick-walled bladder and bilateral hydroureter and hydronephrosis	Abnormal prenatal sonogram Failure to thrive Urinary tract infections	Posterior urethral valves	Associated with severe loss of parenchyma from long-standing hydronephrosis, urine ascites, and urinoma
Neonate with bilateral enlarged echogenic kidneys (echogenic from innumerable tiny cysts) Discrete cysts rarely noted	Abnormal antenatal sonogram or palpable abdominal masses in neonate Anuria Potter's facies	ARPKD	Lethal finding (Potter's syndrome type II)
Multiple bilateral cysts of varying sizes Cysts may also be noted in liver	Palpable abdominal masses in neonate	ADPKD	Rare in neonates and children May appear similar to ARPKD

Multiple cysts of varying size; usually unilateral, may be bilateral Hydronephrosis may be present	Abnormal antenatal sonogram Palpable abdominal mass(es) in neonate Anuria if bilateral	Multicystic dysplastic kidney	Bilateral finding is lethal (Potter's syndrome type II)
Large heterogenous mass within kidney Sharp parenchymal interface with a hypoechoic rim Color Doppler imaging demonstrates flow around mass and some flow within mass	Palpable abdominal mass Hematuria Pain Fever	Wilms' tumor (nephroblastoma) Mesoblastic nephroma	Malignancy: tumor extension into renal vein and IVC, enlarged lymph nodes, metastases Associated with sporadic aniridia, Beckwith-Wiedemann syndrome, hemihypertrophy *continued*

Pediatric Studies—*cont'd*

Sonographic Finding(s)	Clinical Presentation	Differential Diagnosis	Next Step
Large echogenic mass usually homogenous; may demonstrate heterogenicity related to areas of hemorrhage or necrosis Color Doppler imaging demonstrates some flow within mass	Palpable abdominal mass in infant	Mesoblastic nephroma Wilms' tumor	Most common renal mass in infants Usually benign
Heterogenous mass; in neonates mass is markedly hypoechoic Calcifications with/without shadowing may be noted Areas of hemorrhage, cystic change or necrosis may be noted	Palpable abdominal mass	Neuroblastoma	Kidney may be difficult to locate if mass is very large May be difficult to differentiate from Wilms' tumor in some cases Metastases to liver may be noted

Color Doppler imaging demonstrates flow around and within mass IVC, aorta, and ipsilateral kidney are displaced			
Cystic mass near porta hepatic (second gallbladder) Dilated intrahepatic ducts may be noted	Jaundice Pain Mass	Choledochal cyst	Large cysts may contain sludge Nuclear medicine imaging confirms diagnosis
Small or absent gallbladder Liver size and echogenicity may be normal or increased If gallbladder is present, lack of contractility after feeding	Jaundice Labs: abnormal LFT	Biliary atresia Neonatal hepatitis	Lack of formation of bile ducts in fetus

continued

Pediatric Studies—*cont'd*

Sonographic Finding(s)	Clinical Presentation	Differential Diagnosis	Next Step
Multiple layers of bowel (multiple rings of bowel walls); noncompressible	Severe abdominal pain Decreased bowel sounds	Intussusception	Graded compression technique Mass causing intussusception may be noted
Cyst in pelvis of newborn, infant, or female child	Cystic structure noted on prenatal sonogram Mass palpated in neonatal abdomen/pelvis Child: precocious puberty	Ovarian cyst Mesenteric duplication cyst Hydrocolpos	Newborn/infant: ovarian cyst should regress when maternal hormonal stimulation is not present
In transverse axis views, spinal cord demonstrates as two cords (split cord)	Tuft of hair noted in sacral region	Diastematomyelia	Associated with myelomeningocele, meningocele, lipoma, dermal sinus, hydromelia, cord tethering

Spina bifida with low termination of spinal cord and sac containing cerebral spinal fluid and nerves	Abnormal prenatal sonogram	Myelomeningocele	Preoperative scan for hydromelia, diastematomyelia, lipoma, thick filum terminale Use care when scanning sac; use sterile transducer cover and sterile cover over sac Associated with presence of Chiari type II malformation
Conus medullaris visualized at L3 or lower; may be eccentrically located Decreased cord oscillations noted	Cutaneous markers: tuft of hair, lipoma, sinus tract, atypical lumbosacral dimples, hemangioma, skin tag, imperforate anus	Tethered cord	Associated with reflex changes, sensory loss, muscle wasting, power loss, sphincter control problems *continued*

Pediatric Studies—*cont'd*

Sonographic Finding(s)	Clinical Presentation	Differential Diagnosis	Next Step
Unilateral or bilateral dilation of ventricular atrium (>8.0 mm) Third ventricle and massa intermedia may be noted Choroid plexus thickness may be decreased Transcranial Doppler imaging may demonstrate a rising RI with increased intracranial pressure	Abnormal prenatal sonogram Preterm or term neonate Known neural tube defect	Ventriculomegaly Communicating Noncommunicating	Ventricle enlargement with increased HC = hydrocephalus Communicating is associated with neural tube defects Noncommunicating is associated with aqueductal stenosis or obstruction by clot
In preterm neonate, moderate to highly echogenic mass at caudothalamic groove	Changes in blood pressure Endotracheal suctioning Sudden drop in hematocrit	SEH IVH	Grade I confined to germinal matrix (SEH) Grade II IVH extends into ventricle

With progression of bleeding, layered echogenic material in occipital horn (choroid may appear "large") Hemorrhage changes appearance with time; echogenicity change with clot retraction	Blood noted in cerebral spinal fluid		Grade III IVH with ventricular dilation (midline displacement may be noted)
Grade IV IVH with evidence of hemorrhage in periventricular region; initially echogenic changing to anechoic Ventricle is dilated and may contain clot Midline displacement may be noted	Decreased hematocrit	Grade IV IVH with IPH	May progress to porencephalic cyst with connection to dilated ventricle

continued

Pediatric Studies—*cont'd*

Sonographic Finding(s)	Clinical Presentation	Differential Diagnosis	Next Step
Single or multiple cysts that communicate with a lateral ventricle Ventricle may be dilated	Preterm neonate with history of hypoxic/ischemic insult, periventricular hemorrhage, infection, birth trauma, ventricular puncture	Porencephalic cyst (sequel of infarct causing loss of brain parenchyma and cavitation or cyst formation)	Associated with developmental delays
Increased echogenicity of parenchyma adjacent to ventricles Progression to anechoic areas of cystic degeneration located in previously noted abnormal echogenic parenchyma	Preterm neonate with history of hypoxic/ischemic insult	PVL; also known as white matter necrosis Grade IV IVH	Normal slight echogenic blush adjacent to ventricles may mimic early PVL Serial sonograms will demonstrate change tissue from echogenic to cyst formation Cysts may communicate with ventricles

Widely separated lateral ventricles (bat-wing appearance) Absence of the cavum septum pellucidum with radiating sulci Third ventricle is noted between lateral ventricles and is enlarged Ventriculomegaly especially in the atria and occipital horns	Abnormal antenatal sonogram	Agenesis of corpus callosum 　Partial 　Complete	Associated with Chiari type II malformation, Dandy-Walker malformation, holoprosencephaly, lipoma of corpus callosum May be isolated finding
Cystic structure in posterior fossa	Abnormal prenatal sonogram	Dandy-Walker malformation Large cisterna magna Posterior fossa cyst	Associated with neural tube defects, trisomies 13, 18, 21, cardiac, GU, and GI anomalies, cystic hygroma An enlarged cisterna magna may be seen with agenesis of the corpus callosum, hypoplastic vermis, and hydrocephalus *continued*

Pediatric Studies—*cont'd*

Sonographic Finding(s)	Clinical Presentation	Differential Diagnosis	Next Step
Midline displacement by hyperechoic mass; calcifications and cystic areas may be noted	Increased HC and intracranial pressure	Teratoma Abscess Glioma	Obstruction of ventricle system may be noted
Widened and echogenic sulci Fluid collections Focal or diffuse increased parenchyma echogenicity	Exposure to *Escherichia coli*, group B streptococci, influenza, *Streptococcus pneumonia*	Meningitis	Associated with development of ventriculitis and noncommunicating ventriculomegaly
Ventricles are slitlike or dilated; septations Thickened, irregular, hyperechoic ependyma and choroid plexus	Complication of meningitis	Ventriculitis	Associated with development of noncommunicating ventriculomegaly

Calcifications are noted in the brain parenchyma	Abnormal prenatal sonogram History of exposure to toxoplasmosis, CMV, rubella, or herpes simplex virus	Calcifications from infection Vascular calcifications	CMV is the most common congenital infection
Caudal displacement of cerebellar hemispheres Partial or complete agenesis of corpus callosum Unable to visualize cisterna magna Hydrocephalus may be noted	Abnormal prenatal sonogram	Chiari type II malformation	Associated with spina bifida, high cervical encephalo-meningomyelocele, or severe hypoplasia of cerebellum
Large midline fluid-filled space with a mantle of brain tissue; falx may or may not be present	Abnormal prenatal sonogram Hypotelorism or cyclopia and proboscis may be noted	Holoprosencephaly Alobar Semilobar Lobar	Associated with clubfoot, omphalocele, IUGR, and features of trisomy 13 or 18, Meckel-Gruber syndrome

continued

Pediatric Studies—*cont'd*

Sonographic Finding(s)	Clinical Presentation	Differential Diagnosis	Next Step
May demonstrate as a univentricle (horseshoe-shaped ventricle) Thalamus appears fused Agenesis of the corpus callosum Ventriculomegaly or hydrocephalus may be present		Septo-optic dysplasia	It may be difficult to differentiate semilobar from alobar holoprosencephaly
Large, fluid-filled cranium with cerebellum and midbrain seen No brain mantle seen	Abnormal prenatal sonogram	Hydranencephaly Massive hydrocephalus	Falx may or may not be intact

In a term newborn absence of convolutional markings; brain appears "smooth" Lateral and third ventricles may be dilated Absent pulsations of MCA in Sylvian fissure Increased periventricular echogenicity	Abnormal prenatal sonogram Dysmorphic facies	Lissencephaly	Most severe form of neuronal migration anomalies Associated with Walker-Warburg syndrome
Midline cystic mass located between lateral ventricles, posterior to foramen of Monroe and superior to the third ventricle	Newborn/infant with congestive heart failure, cyanosis, and seizures Increased head circumference if hydrocephalus is present	Vein of Galen malformation/aneurysm	Must be differentiated from parenchymal arteriovenous malformation *continued*

Pediatric Studies—*cont'd*

Sonographic Finding(s)	Clinical Presentation	Differential Diagnosis	Next Step
Color Doppler imaging demonstrates flow in the mass Hydrocephalus, calcifications, and brain atrophy may be noted	Child: headaches and seizures		
Proximal femur moves more than 6.0 mm on right or 4.0 mm on left during stress maneuvers but cannot be displaced out of acetabulum (subluxable)	Family history of development dysplasia of hip Breech position, oligohydramnios, and first pregnancy (all may limit mobility of hips in utero)	Unstable hip Subluxable Dislocatable Dislocate	Hips will demonstrate normal movement within acetabulum with stress maneuvers Instability may resolve without treatment

Proximal femur can be displaced out of acetabulum but can be reduced (dislocatable)
Proximal femur is displaced out of acetabulum and cannot be reduced (dislocated)
Acetabulum may appear flattened or shallow

Female infant
Visual inspection notes asymmetric skin folds and shortening of affected thigh

Audible click heard during Ortolani maneuver does not imply dysplasia

MISCELLANEOUS

Chapter 17 Miscellaneous

Miscellaneous

Application	Procedure Information
Baker's cyst	Cystic structure posterior to knee Noticed as swelling or pain Differential diagnosis: popliteal aneurysm, venous thrombophlebitis
TIPS (decompression of the portal system in cases of severe portal hypertension)	2D imaging demonstrates the shunt as a corrugated tubular structure extending from the portal vein to the hepatic vein. Color Doppler imaging demonstrates patency of the shunt. Spectral Doppler analysis of the portal vein, hepatic artery, shunt (proximal, mid, distal), hepatic veins, IVC, and splenic vein. PSV in the shunt: 73–185 cm/s; compare with baseline postoperative examination Decreased portal flow with shunt failure; hepatic artery flow increases with increased RI (>0.6).
Liver transplant	Baseline (within 24 hours of surgery) 2D evaluation of liver and biliary system, color and spectral Doppler of the hepatic artery and portal vein should be performed. Ascites and perihepatic fluid collections are common.

Complications include infection, vascular thrombosis (hepatic artery, portal vein), stenosis or anastomosis leakage, bile duct stricture or stenosis, bilomas, hematomas, renal dysfunction, and recurrence of original disease.

Rejection: fever, malaise, anorexia, hepatomegaly, elevated bilirubin, ALP, and serum transaminase.

Hepatic artery thrombosis (absent signal) may be noted along with parenchymal changes.

Hepatic artery stenosis: PSV >200 cm/s with poststenotic turbulence and color Doppler aliasing or distal to stenosis: systolic acceleration time >0.8, RI <0.5.

IVC stenosis or thrombosis is uncommon complications.

Renal transplant	Baseline (within 24 hours of surgery) 2D evaluation of the kidney with measurements, color and spectral Doppler imaging of the renal artery and vein, and color Doppler assessment of the renal parenchyma should be performed
	Complications include parenchymal pathology (ATN, acute/chronic rejection, infection), prerenal (vascular flow to and from kidney), and postrenal (intrinsic or extrinsic lesions causing obstruction of the ureter)

continued

Miscellaneous—*cont'd*	
Application	Procedure Information
	ATN and acute rejection: increase in kidney size, decreased cortical thickness, increased or decreased cortical echogenicity, loss of corticomedullary differentiation and renal sinus echoes, prominent renal pyramids. Color and spectral Doppler findings may be normal or demonstrate diffuse decreased flow; RI is nonspecific.
	Chronic rejection appears similar to chronic renal failure in the native kidneys
	Infections include pyelonephritis, emphysematous pyelonephritis, pyonephrosis, and abscess
	Renal artery thrombosis: absence of blood flow; related to acute rejection
	Renal artery stenosis in the donor or recipient portions or at the anastomosis. PSV >200 cm/s with poststenotic turbulence. False positive may be due to compression of renal artery during scan!
	Renal vein thrombosis causes swelling of the allograft and abrupt cessation of renal function. Spectral and color Doppler imaging demonstrate absence of flow within main renal vein with reversal of diastolic flow in renal artery
	Renal vein stenosis demonstrates as a region of focal high-velocity turbulent flow

Ureter obstruction can be caused by a stricture at the anastomosis site, by an intraluminal lesion, or by extrinsic compression

Harmonic imaging is ideal for imaging the collecting system

Arteriovenous malformations and pseudoaneurysms may result post biopsy of the allograft

Perinephric fluid collections include hematoma, urinoma, and lymphocele

Pancreas transplant	Baseline (within 24 hours of surgery) 2D evaluation of the pancreas; sonographer must know the surgical technique used for the transplant. Transplants are located in the right lower quadrant (systemic venous-bladder drainage) or right upper quadrant (portal venous-enteric drainage). Examination of the transplanted pancreas is complicated by overlying bowel gas Complications include vascular thrombosis, graft thrombosis, arteriovenous fistula, rejection (increased RI), pancreatitis, fluid collections, and bowel obstruction
Ultrasound guided biopsy/drainage	Needle tip must be at angle to sound beam; needle-guide transducer attachments may be used or the needle may be inserted freehand

continued

Miscellaneous—*cont'd*	
Application	**Procedure Information**
	Sonographic needles or roughened needle tips improve visualization of needle during procedure. Deep biopsies or aspirations require thicker needles than more superficial procedures. A biopsy "gun" or spring-loaded needle may used by the physician. The sonographer should have an assortment of needles and ancillary equipment available for the physician
	Sterile procedures should be followed. The sonographer may assist in the set up an appropriate biopsy or fluid aspiration/removal tray. The sonographer may assist the physician by scanning the area of interest from outside the sterile field or by scanning within the sterile field (sterile transducer cover and gel should be used).
	The sonographer should follow the instructions of the physician during the procedure.

APPENDIXES

American College of Radiology: *ACR practice guideline for the performance of diagnostic and screening ultrasound of the abdominal aorta, neurosonology in neonates and young children, ultrasound examination for detection of developmental dysplasia of the hip, a thyroid and parathyroid ultrasound examination, a breast ultrasound examination, an ultrasound examination of the abdomen and/or retroperitoneum, pelvic ultrasound in females, antepartum obstetrical ultrasound, ultrasound evaluation of the prostate (and surrounding structures), and scrotal ultrasound examinations,* Reston, VA, 2006, American College of Radiology.

American College of Radiology: *ACR practice guideline for performing and interpreting diagnostic ultrasound examinations,* Reston, VA, 2006, American College of Radiology.

American Institute of Ultrasound in Medicine: *AIUM practice guideline for the performance of an antepartum obstetric ultrasound examination,* Laurel, MD, 2003, AIUM.

American Institute of Ultrasound in Medicine: *AIUM practice guideline for the performance of a thyroid and parathyroid ultrasound examination,* Laurel, MD, 2003, AIUM.

American Institute of Ultrasound in Medicine: *AIUM practice guideline for the performance of the ultrasound examination for detection of developmental dysplasia of the hip,* Laurel, MD, 2003, AIUM.

American Institute of Ultrasound in Medicine: *AIUM practice guideline for the performance of the breast ultrasound examination,* Laurel, MD, 2002, AIUM.

American Institute of Ultrasound in Medicine: *AIUM practice guideline for the performance of diagnostic and screening ultrasound examinations of the abdominal aorta,* Laurel, MD, 2006, AIUM.

American Institute of Ultrasound in Medicine: *AIUM practice guideline for the performance of neurosonology in neonates and young children,* Laurel, MD, 2006, AIUM.

American Institute of Ultrasound in Medicine: *AIUM standard for the performance of an ultrasound examination of the abdomen or retroperitoneum,* Laurel, MD, 2006, AIUM.

American Institute of Ultrasound in Medicine: *AIUM practice guideline for the performance of an ultrasound examination of the female pelvis,* Laurel, MD, 2006, AIUM.

American Institute of Ultrasound in Medicine: *AIUM practice guideline for the performance of ultrasound evaluation of the prostate and surrounding structures,* Laurel, MD, 2006, AIUM.

American Institute of Ultrasound in Medicine: *AIUM practice guideline for the performance of scrotal ultrasound examinations,* Laurel, MD, 2006, AIUM.

American Institute of Ultrasound in Medicine: *Standard presentation and labeling of ultrasound images A stage 2 standard,* Laurel, MD, 2006, AIUM.

Bates-Tempkin B: Ultrasound scanning principles and protocols, ed 2, St. Louis, 1999, WB Saunders.

Callen P: *Ultrasonography in obstetrics and gynecology,* ed 4, St. Louis, 2000, WB Saunders.

Coffin C, editor: *Ultrasound examination guidelines,* Dallas, 2000, Society of Diagnostic Medical Sonographers.

Craig M: *Essentials of sonography and patient care,* ed 2, St. Louis, 2006, WB Saunders.

Curry R, Bates-Tempkin B: *Ultrasonography: an introduction to normal structure and function,* ed 2, St. Louis, 2004, W B Saunders.

Daigle R: *National certification examination review vascular technology,* ed 3, Dallas, 2004, Society of Diagnostic Medical Sonography.

Fatchett J: Basic abdominal sonography procedural overview, *J Diag Med Sonography Suppl* 13:24s–28s, 1997.

Green L, editor: *Abdominal ultrasound protocol manual,* St. Pete Beach, 2004, Gulfcoast Ultrasound Institute.

Green L, editor: *Gynecological ultrasound protocol manual,* St. Pete Beach, 2004, Gulfcoast Ultrasound Institute.

Green L, editor: *Obstetrical ultrasound protocol manual,* St. Pete Beach, 2004, Gulfcoast Ultrasound Institute.

Hagen-Ansert S: *Textbook of diagnostic ultrasonography,* ed 6, St. Louis, 2006, Mosby.

Henningsen C: *National certification examination review obstetrics and gynecology,* ed 3, Dallas, 2004, Society of Diagnostic Medical Sonography.

Nyberg D et al: *Diagnostic imaging of fetal anomalies,* Philadelphia, 2003, Lippincott.

Rumack C et al: *Diagnostic ultrasound,* ed 3, St. Louis, 2005, Mosby.

Siegel M: *Pediatric sonography,* ed 3, Philadelphia, 2002, Lippincott.

Weinberg K: *National certification examination review abdomen,* ed 3, Dallas, 2004, Society of Diagnostic Medical Sonography.

References for Protocols and Practices

Appendix B References for Sonographic Measurements

Curry R, Bates-Tempkin B: *Ultrasonography: an introduction to normal structure and function,* ed 2, St. Louis, 2004, WB Saunders.

Daigle R: *National certification examination review: Vascular technology,* ed 3, Dallas, 2004, Society of Diagnostic Medical Sonography.

Goldberg B, McGahan J: *Atlas of ultrasound measurements,* ed 2, St. Louis, 2006, Mosby.

Hagen-Ansert S: *Textbook of diagnostic ultrasonography,* ed 6, St. Louis, 2006, Mosby.

Hennerici M et al: *Vascular diagnosis with ultrasound,* ed 2, New York, 2006, Thieme.

Henningsen C: *Clinical guide to ultrasonography,* St. Louis, 2004, Mosby.

Henningsen C: *National certification examination review: obstetrics and gynecology,* ed 3, 2004, Dallas, Society of Diagnostic Medical Sonography.

Hricak H et al: *Pocket radiologist: gynecology top 100 diagnoses,* Salt Lake City, 2004, Amirsys.

McGahan J, Goldberg B: *Diagnostic ultrasound: a logical approach,* Philadelphia, 1998, Lippincott.

Middleton W et al: *The requisites: ultrasound,* ed 2, St. Louis, 2004, Mosby.

Rumack C et al: *Diagnostic ultrasound,* ed 3, St. Louis, 2005, Mosby.

Sanders R, Winter T: *Clinical sonography: a practical guide,* ed 4, Philadelphia, 2007, Lippincott.

Siegel M: *Pediatric sonography,* ed 3, Philadelphia, 2002, Lippincott.

Weinberg K: *National certification examination review: abdomen,* ed 3, Dallas, 2004, Society of Diagnostic Medical Sonography.

Woodward P et al: *Diagnostic imaging: obstetrics,* Salt Lake City, 2005, Amirsys.

Routine Blood Chemistry

Test	Normal Values	SI Units
Glucose, fasting (FBS)		
Infant		
Child <2 years	40–90 mg/dl	2.2–5 mmol/L
Child >2	60–100 mg/dl	3.3–5.5 mmol/L
years-adult	70–105 mg/dl	3.9–5.8 mmol/L
Proteins		
Total	6.4–8.3 g/dl	64–83 g/L
Albumin	3.5–5 g/dl	35–50 g/L
Globulin	2–3.5 g/dl	20–35 g/L
Albumin/	1.5:1–2.5:1	1.5:1–2.5:1
globulin ratio		

continued

Routine Blood Chemistry—*cont'd*

Test	Normal Values	SI Units
BUN		
Child	5–18 mg/dl	
Adult	10–20 mg/dl	3.6–7.1 mmol/L
Creatinine		
Infant	0.2–0.4 mg/dl	
Child	0.3–0.7 mg/dl	
Adult	0.5–1.2 mg/dl	44–106 µmol/L
Calcium	9–11 mg/dl	2.25–2.74 mmol/L
Bilirubin		
Total	0.3–1 mg/dl	5.1–17 µmol/L
Indirect	0.2–0.8 mg/dl	3.4–12 µmol/L
Direct	0.1–0.3 mg/dl	1.7–5.1 µmol/L
AST/SGOT	0–35 units/L	0–0.58 µkat/L

ALP		
Child	60–300 units/L	
Adult	30–120 units/L	0.5–2 µkat/L
ALT/SGPT	4–36 international units/ L@37° C	4–36 units/L
Sodium	136–145 mEq/L	136–145 mmol/L
Potassium	3.5–5 mEq/L	3.5–5 mmol/L
Chloride	98–106 mEq/L	98–106 mmol/L
CO_2	23–30 mEq/L	23–30 mmol/L
Magnesium	1.3–2.1 mEq/L	0.65–1.05 mmol/L

From Pagana KD, Pagana TJ: *Mosby's manual of diagnostic laboratory tests*, ed 2, St. Louis, 2002, Mosby.

Normal Lab Values

Complete Blood Cell Count With Differential

Test	Normal Values	SI Units
WBCs	5,000–10,000/mm^3	5–10 × 10^9/L
RBCs		
Male	4.7–6.1 × 10^6/μL	4.7–6.1 × 10^{12}/L
Female	4.2–5.4 × 10^6/μL	4.2–5.4 × 10^{12}/L
Hgb		
Child (varies)	10–15 g/dl	
Male	14–18 g/dl	8.7–11.2 mmol/L
Female	12–16 g/dl	7.4–9.9 mmol/L
HCT		
Child (varies)	29%–44%	
Male	42%–52%	0.42–0.52
Female	37%–47%	0.37–0.47

MCV	82–98 fL	82–98 fL
MCH	27–33 pg	27–33 pg
MCHC	32%–36%	0.32–0.36
RDW	10.2%–14.5%	10.2%–14.5%
WBC diff		
Neutrophils	55%–70%	0.55–0.70
Lymphocytes	20%–40%	0.20–0.40
Monocytes	2%–8%	0.02–0.08
Eosinophils	1%–4%	0.01–0.04
Basophils	0.5%–1%	0.005–0.01
Plt count	150,000–400,000/mm3	$150–400 \times 10^9/L$

continued

Complete Blood Cell Count With Differential—*cont'd*

Test	Normal Values	SI Units
RBC morphology (RBC smear)	Normal size, shape, color	
RBC	Normal quantity	
RBC, WBC, Plt	Normal count	
WBC diff		

From Pagana KD, Pagana TJ: *Mosby's manual of diagnostic laboratory tests*, ed 2, St. Louis, 2002, Mosby.

Coagulation Studies

Test	Normal Values	SI Units
Bleeding time (Ivy method)	3–9.5 min	180–570 sec
PT	10–14 sec	10–14 sec
INR	2–3.5	2–3.5
PPT	60–70 sec	60–70 sec
APPT	30–40 sec	30–40 sec
TT	8–12 sec	8–12 sec
Fibrinogen	200–400 mg/dl	2–4 g/L
Plasminogen	2.4–4.4 CTA units/ml	

continued

Coagulation Studies—*cont'd*

Test	Normal Values	SI Units
Pit count (Thrombocyte count)	150,000–400,000/mm^3	150–400 × 10^9/L
MPV	7.4–10.4 fL	

From Pagana KD, Pagana TJ: *Mosby's manual of diagnostic laboratory tests*, ed 2, St. Louis, 2002, Mosby.

Hepatic Function Panel

Test	Normal Values	SI Units
Albumin	3.5–5 g/dl	35–50 g/L
Bilirubin, total	0.3–1 mg/dl	5.1–17 µmol/L
Bilirubin, indirect	0.2–0.8 mg/dl	3.4–12 µmol/L
Bilirubin, direct	0.1–.03 mg/dl	1.7–5.1 µmol/L
Alkaline phosphatase Child Adult	 60–300 units/L 30–120 units/L	 0.5–2 µkat/L

continued

Hepatic Function Panel—*cont'd*

Test	Normal Values	SI Units
ALT/SGPT	4–36 international units/L	4–36 units/L
AST	0–35 units/L	0–0.58 μkat/L
Protein, total	6.4–8.3 g/dl	64–83 g/L

From Pagana KD, Pagana TJ: *Mosby's manual of diagnostic laboratory tests*, ed 2, St. Louis, 2002, Mosby.

Lipid Panel

Test	Normal Values	SI Units
Total cholesterol	<200 mg/dl (age dependent)	<5.20 mmol/L
HDLs		
Male	>45 mg/dl	>0.75 mmol/L
Female	>55 mg/dl	>0.91 mmol/L
LDLs	60–180 mg/dl	<3.37 mmol/L
VLDLs	25%–50%	
Triglycerides		
Male	40–160 mg/dl	0.45–1.81 mmol/L
Female	35–135 mg/dl	0.40–1.52 mmol/L

From Pagana KD, Pagana TJ: *Mosby's manual of diagnostic laboratory tests*, ed 2, St. Louis, 2002, Mosby.

Thyroid Panel

Test	Normal Values	SI Units
T_4	5–12 mcg/dl	64–154 nmol/L
FT_4	0.8–2.3 ng/dl	10–30 pmol/L
T_3 uptake	25%–35%	0.25–0.35
Total T_3	110–230 ng/dl	1.7–3.5 nmol/L
TSH	0.3–5.4 microunits/ml	0.3–5.4 milliunits/L

Lewis SM, Heitkemper MM, Dirksen SR: *Medical-surgical nursing: assessment and management of clinical problems*, ed 6, St Louis, 2003, Mosby.

Urinalysis

Test	Normal Values
Appearance	Clear
Color	Straw/amber
Odor	Aromatic
pH	4.6–8
Protein	Negative
Specific gravity	1.005–1.030

continued

Urinalysis—*cont'd*

Test	Normal Values
Glucose	Negative
Casts	None
WBCs	0–4
RBCs	<2

24-Hour Urine Chemistry

Test	Normal Values	SI Units
Amylase	6.5–48.1 units/hr	
Calcium	100–250 mg/day	2.5–6.3 mmol/day
Chloride		
Child	15–40 mmol/day	
Adult	110–250 mEq/day	110–250 mmol/day
Creatinine		
Child 1.5–7 yr	10–15 mg/kg/day	
Child 7–15 yr	5.2–41 mg/kg/day	
Adult	0.8–2 g/day	7.1–17.7 mmol/day

continued

24-Hour Urine Chemistry—*cont'd*

Test	Normal Values	SI Units
Creatinine clearance	85–135 ml/min	1.42–2.25 ml/sec
Magnesium	5–10 mEq/day	
Potassium	25–100 mEq/L/day	25–100 mmol/day
Sodium	40–220 mEq/L/day	40–220 mmol/day
Uric acid	250–750 mg/day	1.48–4.43 mmol/day

Abdominal Aorta

- Suprarenal: low resistance, no spectral broadening
- Infrarenal: high resistance with possible triphasic signal distally
- PSV at level of renal arteries: 70–140 cm/s

Inferior Vena Cava

- Pulsatile flow proximally; phasic flow distally; wide spectrum of flow

Celiac Trunk

- Low resistance, constant forward flow
- PSV: 50–160 cm/s; EDV < 50 cm/s spectral broadening from tortuous vessel

Common Hepatic Artery

- Low resistance flow
- PSV: <100 cm/s

Splenic Artery

- Low resistance, turbulent flow
- PSV: <200 cm/s; spectral broadening from vessel tortuosity

Hepatic Vein

- Same waveform as IVC; pulsatile flow pattern dependent on cardiac cycle and pressures in right atrium

Superior Mesenteric Artery

- Fasting: high resistance; PSV: <275 cm/s
- Postprandial: low resistance; increased systolic flow; diastolic flow should double

Portal Veins

- Undulating flow pattern caused by effects of respiration
- Continuous flow with low peak and mean velocities
- Affected by posture, exercise (decreased flow), and dietary state (eating = increased flow); use supine or left lateral

decubitus position after 8 hours of fasting to reduce variations in flow

Main Renal Artery

- Low resistance flow with low pulsatility; constant diastolic flow; spectral broadening
- PSV: <120 cm/s; RI: 0.58–0.7; RAR: <3.5
- Acceleration time: 0.07–0.1 s; acceleration index: >3.78
- S/D ratio: >0.23
- Renal artery duplication is common

Intrarenal Artery

- Dampened signal with reduced velocity compared with main renal artery
- RI: 0.7 (not accurate for patients under the age of 6 years and the elderly)

Renal Vein

- Low-velocity continuous signal

Common Iliac Arteries

- High resistance, triphasic waveform

Common Iliac Vein

- Continuous low-flow signal; pulsations from adjacent artery may be noted

Ovarian Artery

- Ovulation: velocity increase; RI: 0.4–0.5
- Preovulatory: high resistance; RI: 0.5–0.6 (resting ovary)

Uterine Artery

- High velocity, high resistance
- Pregnancy: low resistance; increased diastolic flow

Testicular Artery

- Low resistance
- Power Doppler imaging is more sensitive to slow flow

Testicular Vein

- Pampiniform plexus should not dilate with Valsalva maneuver

Extremity Arteries

- High resistance, triphasic waveform in resting state; low resistance in response to exercise

Extremity Veins

- Continuous low flow; vessel walls can be coapted

Thyroid Artery

- PSV in major arteries: 20.0–40.0 cm/s
- PSV in intraparenchymal arteries: 15.0–30.0 cm/s

Pregnancy

- Umbilical artery: S/D ratio; RI: normal high resistance in nongravid uterus changes to low resistance during pregnancy
- Umbilical vein: pulsations in early pregnancy decreasing to a continuous waveform in late pregnancy
- Fetal middle cerebral artery: high systolic velocity and low diastolic velocity; PI may be obtained

- Ovarian torsion may occur because of the laxity of ligaments during pregnancy; surgical intervention may be required.
- Hydronephrosis is a common occurrence, especially the right kidney; stent placement may be required to maintain patency of the ureter.
- Cystitis is common and may cause uterine irritation and contractions that mimics preterm labor.
- Cholelithiasis occurs commonly in pregnant women; surgery may be required.
- Appendicitis is not uncommon and may mimic ectopic pregnancy; surgery may be required.
- Hyperemesis may cause dehydration and possible maternal weight loss; it may be related to abnormally high β–human chorionic gonadotropin levels.
- Maternal cyanotic congenital heart disease may cause a decrease in oxygen to the fetus (underlying cause of placental insufficiency).
- Viral infections such as cytomegalovirus, herpes, chickenpox, rubella, influenza, or human immunodeficiency virus infection/acquired immunodeficiency syndrome may affect the fetal neural tube, heart, growth (intrauterine growth restriction [IUGR]), liver, and the amount of amniotic fluid.
- Bacterial infections such as urinary tract infection, gonorrhea, or syphilis may affect the placenta, fetal brain, and growth (IUGR) and may cause fetal death.
- Parasitic infections such as toxoplasmosis and malaria may affect fetal growth (IUGR), brain, and liver and may cause fetal death.
- Endocrine/metabolic diseases such as diabetes, hyperthyroidism or hypothyroidism and hyperparathyroidism affect the placenta; fetal growth (IUGR), brain, or heart and may cause fetal goiter or death.
- Hematological diseases such as isoimmunization (Rh incompatibility), sickle cell anemia, and thalassemia affect

fetal growth (IUGR) and amniotic fluid volume and may cause hydrops fetalis.

- Systemic lupus erythematosus is a multisystem autoimmune disease. Antibodies may cross the placenta and cause toxemia, recurrent abortion, IUGR, and fetal death. Pregnancy may be successful if planned during a time when this disease is controlled.
- Maternal hypertension (chronic, essential, or pregnancy-induced) increases the risk of stillbirth, preeclampsia, IUGR, placental abruption, small placenta, and oligohydramnios.
- Toxemia of pregnancy: Preeclampsia to severe preeclampsia leads to the development of hypertension, proteinuria, and edema and affects fetal growth (IUGR). Untreated or uncontrolled seizures, coma, and death (eclampsia) may occur.
- Teratogenic effects of drug use depend on the type of drug, dosage, time of exposure, host susceptibility, period of gestation, and so forth. Abused drugs include alcohol, amphetamines, barbiturates, narcotics, nicotine, and caffeine. Drug use is associated with a wide range of fetal anomalies.
- Malnutrition: Low maternal weight may be related to drug use; the fetus is at risk for IUGR or central nervous system abnormalities.
- Malnutrition: Obesity increases the maternal risk of hypertension, severe preeclampsia, multiple gestation, and gestational diabetes; it may require a cesarean section delivery. The fetus is at risk for neural tube defects.
- Maternal diabetes may predate the pregnancy or only manifest during pregnancy (gestational diabetes). Complications include poor glucose control and serious maternal infections. The risk of macrosomia or IUGR (in diabetic patients with vascular compromise), unexplained stillbirth, congenital anomalies (caudal regression, heart defects, neural tube defects), and polyhydramnios is increased in diabetic pregnancies.

Greetings and Instructions

Hello, my name is _____. *Buenos días, me llamo _____.*

I will be performing your ultrasound examination. *Estaré realizando su examen de ultrasonido.*

What is your name? *Como se llama?*

Please come with me. *Favor de venire conmigo.*

Please remove all clothing and put on the gown. *Favor de quitar toda su ropy y ponga la bata.*

Please remove your clothing below the waist and put on the gown. *Favor de quitar su ropa debajo de la cintura.*

Please remove your clothing above the waist and put on the gown. *Favor de quitar su ropa arriba de la cintura.*

Are you too cold or too hot? *Tiene demasiado frío o demasiado caliente? Calor?*

Patient Preparation

When was the last time you ate food or drank water? *Cuando era la última vez que comió o tomo alimento o agua?*

How much water did you drink? *Que cantidad de agua tomo?*

Patient History

What medicine are you taking? *Que medicina toma?*

Are you in pain? *Tiene dolor?*

What kind of pain is it? *Que tipo de dolor tiene?*
- Dull/sharp? *sordo/agudo?*
- Throbbing/constant? *palpitante/constante?*
- On and off? *que va y viene?*

Where is your pain? *Donde esta su dolor?*

Are you pregnant? *Esta embarazada?*

How many times have you been pregnant? *Cuantas veces ha estado embarazada?*

How many babies were born alive? *Cuantos bebés nacion vivas?*

What was the date of your last menstrual period? *Cuando fue el primer día de su ultima regla?*

When are you due? *Cuando esta usted debido?*
What is your due date? *Que es su debido data?*
Are you bleeding? *Tiene sangrado? or Esta sangrado?*
There is an 85% chance of a boy/girl. *La probabilidad de que sea una nino/nina es 85 por cien.*

Positioning and Scanning

Please lie down on the table. *Favor de acostarse en la mesa.*
Please turn over on your side. *Favor de acostarse de lado.*
Breathe deeply. *Respire profundo.*
Lift your arms. *Levante los brazos.*
When I tell you, hold your breath. *Cuando le aviso, aguante la respiración.*

Stop breathing. *Aguante la respiracion.*
You can breathe now. *Ya puede respirar ahora.*
Do not move. *No se mueva.*

Ending the Examination

I am finished. That is all. *Yo termine. Es todo.*
I will return shortly. *Refresarse en seguida.*
Remain here. *Quedese aqui.*
Please sit here. *Sientese aqu por favor.*
Now you can get dressed. *Ahora se puede ponar su ropa.*
Your doctor will tell you the results of this test. *Su médico le dirá los resultados de esta prueba.*
Thank you. Goodbye. *Gracias. Adios.*

Glossary of Abbreviations

+ positive
− negative
β beta
2D two-dimensional (gray scale)
3D three-dimensional
AC abdominal circumference
AChE acetylcholinesterase
ACKD acquired cystic kidney disease
ADPKD autosomal dominant polycystic kidney disease
AFP alpha-fetoprotein
AI acceleration index
AIDS acquired immunodeficiency syndrome
ALARA as low as reasonably achievable
ALP alkaline phosphatase
ALT alanine aminotransferase
AP anteroposterior
ARPKD autosomal recessive polycystic kidney disease
ASD atrial septal defect
AST aspartate aminotransferase

ATN acute tubular necrosis
β–hCG beta subunit of human chorionic gonadotropin
BPD biparietal diameter
BUN blood urea nitrogen
BPH benign prostatic hypertrophy
c/o complains of
Ca cancer
CAM cystic adenomatoid malformation
CBD common bile duct
CHD common hepatic duct
CHF congestive heart failure
CI cephalic index
CMV cytomegalovirus
CNS central nervous system
CRL crown-rump length
CT computed tomography
DA diamniotic
DZ dizygotic
EDV end-diastolic velocity

EHD extrahepatic duct
EHR embryonic heart rate
ERCP endoscopic retrograde cholangiopancreatography
ETOH ethanol (alcohol)
EV endovaginal
FHR fetal heart rate
FL femur length
FNH focal nodular hyperplasia
FSH follicle-stimulating hormone
FTT failure to thrive
FUO fever of unknown origin
GA gestational age
GB gallbladder
GFR glomerular filtration rate
GI gastrointestinal
GU genitourinary
HC head circumference
HCC hepatocellular carcinoma

HELLP hemolysis, elevated liver enzymes, low platelets
HRT hormone replacement therapy
IPH intraparenchymal hemorrhage
IUCD/IUD intrauterine contraceptive device
IUP intrauterine pregnancy
IVC inferior vena cava
IVH intraventricular hemorrhage
IVP intravenous pyelogram
LDH lactate dehydrogenase
LEEP loop electrosurgical excision procedure
LFT liver function tests
LGA large for gestational age
LUS lower uterine segment
MA menstrual age
MCDK multicystic dysplastic kidney
MI mechanical index
mIU milli-international unit
MPD main pancreatic duct

Glossary of Abbreviations

MPV main portal vein
MSAFP maternal serum alpha-fetoprotein
MSD mean sac diameter
MZ monozygotic
NT nuchal translucency
OHS/OHSS ovarian hyperstimulation syndrome
PAP Papanicolaou smear/test
PAPP-A pregnancy-associated plasma protein A
PI pulsatility index
PID pelvic inflammatory disease
PROM premature rupture of membranes
PSA prostate-specific antigen
PSV peak systolic velocity
PVL periventricular leukomalacia
RAR renal/aorta ratio
RCC renal cell carcinoma
RI resistive index

RLQ right lower quadrant
RUQ right upper quadrant
SCC squamous cell carcinoma
S/D ratio systolic/diastolic ratio
SEH subependymal hemorrhage
SGA small for gestational age
SMA superior mesenteric artery
STD sexually transmitted disease
T3 tri-iodothyronine
T4 thyroxine
TA transabdominal
TAPVR total anomalous pulmonary venous return
TB tuberculosis
TCC transitional cell carcinoma
TE tracheoesophageal
TES twin embolization syndrome
TGC time gain compensation

TI thermal index
TRAP twin reversed arterial perfusion
TSH thyroid-stimulating hormone
TTTS twin-to-twin transfusion syndrome
UPJ ureteropelvic junction
UTI urinary tract infection
UVJ ureterovesical junction

VACTERL vertebral defects, anal atresia, cardiac malformations, tracheoesophageal fistula, renal anomalies, limb malformation
VATER vertebral defects, anal atresia, tracheoesophageal fistula, renal anomalies
VSD ventricular septal defect
WBC white blood cells

Bibliography

American College of Radiology: *ACR practice guideline for the performance of diagnostic and screening ultrasound of the abdominal aorta, neurosonology in neonates and young children, ultrasound examination for detection of developmental dysplasia of the hip, a thyroid and parathyroid ultrasound examination, a breast ultrasound examination, an ultrasound examination of the abdomen and/or retroperitoneum, pelvic ultrasound in females, antepartum obstetrical ultrasound, ultrasound evaluation of the prostate (and surrounding structures), and scrotal ultrasound examinations,* Reston, VA, 2006, American College of Radiology.

American College of Radiology: *ACR practice guideline for performing and interpreting diagnostic ultrasound examinations,* Reston, VA, 2006, American College of Radiology.

American Institute of Ultrasound in Medicine: *AIUM practice guideline for the performance of the breast ultrasound examination,* Laurel, MD, 2002, AIUIM.

American Institute of Ultrasound in Medicine: *AIUM standard for the performance of an ultrasound examination of the abdomen or retroperitoneum,* Laurel, MD, 2002, AIUM.

American Institute of Ultrasound in Medicine: *AIUM practice guideline for the performance of an antepartum obstetric ultrasound examination* Laurel., MD, 2003, AIUM.

American Institute of Ultrasound in Medicine: *AIUM practice guideline for the performance of a thyroid and parathyroid ultrasound examination,* Laurel, MD, 2003, AIUM.

American Institute of Ultrasound in Medicine: *AIUM practice guideline for the performance of the ultrasound examination for detection of developmental dysplasia of the hip,* Laurel, MD, 2003, AIUM.

American Institute of Ultrasound in Medicine: *AIUM practice guideline for the performance of diagnostic and screening ultrasound Examinations of the abdominal aorta,* Laurel, MD, 2006, AIUM.

American Institute of Ultrasound in Medicine: *AIUM practice guideline for the performance of neurosonology in neonates and young children,* Laurel, MD, 2006, AIUM.

American Institute of Ultrasound in Medicine: *AIUM practice guideline for the performance of scrotal ultrasound examinations,* Laurel, MD, 2006, AIUM.

American Institute of Ultrasound in Medicine: *AIUM practice guideline for the performance of an ultrasound examination of the female pelvis,* Laurel, MD, 2006, AIUM.

American Institute of Ultrasound in Medicine: *AIUM practice guideline for the performance of ultrasound evaluation of the prostate and surrounding structures,* Laurel, MD, 2006, AIUM.

American Institute of Ultrasound in Medicine: *Standard presentation and labeling of ultrasound images, a stage 2 standard,* Laurel, MD, 2006, AIUM.

Bates-Tempkin B: *Ultrasound scanning principles and protocols,* ed e, St. Louis, 1999, WB Saunders.

Benson C et al: *Ultrasonography in obstetrics and gynecology: a practical approach,* New York, 2000, Thieme.

Bisset R, Khan A: *Differential diagnosis in abdominal ultrasound,* ed 2, St. Louis, 2002, WB Saunders.

Callen P: *Ultrasonography in obstetrics and gynecology,* ed 4, St. Louis, 2000, WB Saunders.

Carr-Hoefer C, Grube J: *National certification examination review: breast ultrasound,* Dallas, 2002, Society of Diagnostic Medical Sonography.

Coffin C, editor: *Ultrasound examination guidelines,* Dallas, 2000, Society of Diagnostic Medical Sonographers.

Craig M: *Essentials of sonography and patient care,* ed 2, St. Louis, 2006, WB Saunders.

Curry R, Bates-Tempkin B: *Ultrasonography: an introduction to normal structure and function,* ed 2, St. Louis, 2004, WB Saunders.

Daigle R: *National certification examination review: vascular technology,* ed 3, Dallas, 2004, Society of Diagnostic Medical Sonography.

Doubilet P, Benson C: *Atlas of ultrasound in obstetrics and gynecology: a multimedia reference,* Philadelphia, 2003, Lippincott.

Fatchett J: Basic abdominal sonography procedural overview, *J Diag Med Sonography Suppl* 13:24s–28s, 1997.

Goldberg B, McGahan J: *Atlas of ultrasound measurements,* ed 2, St. Louis, 2006, Mosby.

Green L, editor: *Abdominal ultrasound protocol manual,* St. Pete Beach, 2004, Gulfcoast Ultrasound Institute.

Green L, editor: *Gynecological ultrasound protocol manual,* St. Pete Beach, 2004, Gulfcoast Ultrasound Institute.

Green L, editor: *Obstetrical ultrasound protocol manual,* St. Pete Beach, 2004, Gulfcoast Ultrasound Institute.

Hagen-Ansert S: *Textbook of diagnostic ultrasonography,* ed 6, St. Louis, 2006, Mosby.

Hall R: *The ultrasound handbook,* ed 3, Philadelphia, 1999, Lippincott.

Hennerici M et al: *Vascular diagnosis with ultrasound,* ed 2, New York, 2006, Thieme.

Henningsen C: *Clinical guide to ultrasonography,* St. Louis, 2004, Mosby.

Henningsen C: *National certification examination review: Obstetrics and gynecology,* ed 3, Dallas, 2004, Society of Diagnostic Medical Sonography.

Bibliography

Hickey J, Goldberg F: *Ultrasound review of the abdomen, male pelvis, small parts,* Philadelphia, 1999, Lippincott.

Hricak H et al: *Pocket radiologist: gynecology top 100 diagnoses,* Salt Lake City, 2004, Amirsys.

Krebs C et al: *Ultrasound atlas of disease processes,* New York, 1993, Appleton & Lange.

Krebs C et al: *Ultrasound atlas of vascular diseases,* New York, 1999, Appleton & Lange.

Krebs C et al: *Review for the ultrasonography examination,* ed 3, New York, 2004, Appleton & Lange.

McGahan J, Goldberg B: *Diagnostic ultrasound: a logical approach,* Philadelphia, 1998, Lippincott.

Middleton W et al: *The requisites: ultrasound,* ed 2, St. Louis, 2004, Mosby.

Moore K, Persaud T: *The developing human: Clinically oriented embryology,* ed 7, St. Louis, 2003, WB Saunders.

Nyberg D et al: *Diagnostic imaging of fetal anomalies,* Philadelphia, 2003, Lippincott.

Peneff C, Swearengin R: *National certification examination review: neurosonology,* Dallas, 2004, Society of Diagnostic Medical Sonography.

Rumack C et al: *Diagnostic ultrasound,* ed 3., St. Louis, 2005, Mosby.

Sanders R et al: *Structural fetal abnormalities: the total picture,* St. Louis, 1996, Mosby.

Sanders R, Winter T: *Clinical sonography: a practical guide,* ed 4, Philadelphia, 2007, Lippincott.

Siegel M: *Pediatric sonography,* ed 3, Philadelphia, 2002, Lippincott.

Tegeler C et al: *Neurosonology,* St. Louis, 1996, Mosby.

Weinberg K: *National certification examination review: abdomen,* ed 3, Dallas, 2004, Society of Diagnostic Medical Sonography.

Woodward P et al: *Pocket radiologist: obstetrics top 100 diagnoses,* Salt Lake City, 2003, Amirsys.

Woodward P et al: *Diagnostic imaging: obstetrics,* Salt Lake City, 2005, Amirsys.

Zweibel W, Sohaey R: *Introduction to ultrasound,* St. Louis, 1998, WB Saunders.

Index